Prostaglandins and Thromboxanes

Butterworths Monographs in Chemistry

Butterworths Monographs in Chemistry is a series of occasional texts by internationally acknowledged specialists, providing authoritative treatment of topics of current significance in chemistry and chemical engineering

Forthcoming titles:

Comprehensive Titration
Coordination Catalysis in Organic Chemistry
Liquids and Liquid Mixtures, Third Edition
Strategy in Organic Synthesis

Butterworths Monographs in Chemistry

Prostaglandins and Thromboxanes

Edited by
Roger F. Newton
Chemical Research Department, Glaxo Group Research,
Ware, Hertfordshire

Stanley M. Roberts
Chemical Research Department, Glaxo Group Research,
Greenford, Middlesex

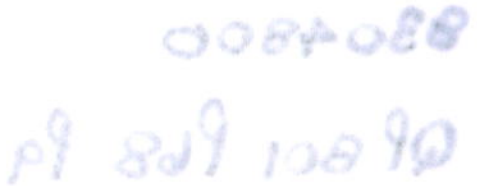

Butterworth Scientific
London Boston Sydney Wellington Durban Toronto

First published 1982

British Library Cataloguing in Publication Data

Prostaglandins and thromboxanes. — (Butterworths monographs in chemistry)
1. Prostaglandins 2. Thromboxanes
I. Roberts, Stanley M. II. Newton, Roger F.
547.7′34 QP801.P68

ISBN 0-408-10773-1

Typeset by Tunbridge Wells Typesetting Services Ltd
Printed and bound in England by Cambridge University Press

Preface

In this book we have collated important information from the biological and physical sciences relating to the preparation and activities of prostaglandins, thromboxanes, and analogues. We are indebted to the Chapter authors for summarizing the vast amount of research work that has been described in the primary literature and presenting it in a way that should be readily assimilated by undergraduates and postgraduates having a sound background in organic chemistry.

It would have been satisfying to report that the research work had already culminated in the discovery, development and marketing of useful clinical drugs. However, the end-products have proved to be somewhat elusive. On the other hand, prostaglandin research is a relatively young science and the charisma and potential of the field have never been greater. Numerous laboratories in industry and academia are presently concentrating their efforts in this direction and new discoveries will doubtless emerge. It is still highly likely that a compound with a structure closely related to a naturally occurring thromboxane or prostaglandin will play a valuable future role in the control of gastric ulceration, thrombosis, arthritis, or another disease state. This breakthrough will owe a lot to the fundamental science described in this text.

Roger F. Newton
Stanley M. Roberts

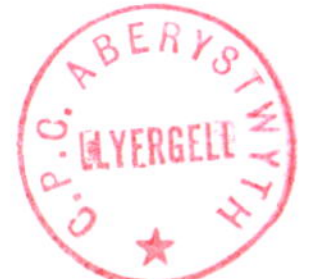

Contributors

Eric W. Collington
Chemical Research Department, Glaxo Group Research, Ware, Hertfordshire

Roger P. Dickinson
Pfizer Central Research, Pfizer Ltd., Sandwich, Kent

Keith H. Gibson
Chemistry Department (II), ICI (Pharmaceuticals) Ltd., Alderley Park, Macclesfield, Cheshire

Ian Kennedy
Department of Pharmacology, Glaxo Group Research, Ware, Hertfordshire

Roger F. Newton
Chemical Research Department, Glaxo Group Research, Ware, Hertfordshire

Stanley M. Roberts
Chemical Research Department, Glaxo Group Research, Greenford, Middlesex

Feodor Scheinmann
Department of Chemistry and Applied Chemistry, University of Salford, Lancashire

Richard J. K. Taylor
School of Chemical Sciences, University of East Anglia, Norwich, Norfolk

Contents

CHAPTER 1

History, nomenclature and potential uses of prostaglandins and thromboxanes in the clinic

Roger F. Newton
Chemical Research Department, Glaxo Group Research, Ware, Hertfordshire

and

Stanley M. Roberts
Chemical Research Department, Glaxo Group Research, Greenford, Middlesex

History

Almost 50 years ago, scientists in Europe and the USA observed that lipid fractions isolated from human semen induced contraction and relaxation of the human uterus. Von Euler coined the name prostaglandin for the active component, erroneously believing that the substance was produced in the prostate gland.

At this time further investigations into the phenomenon were hampered by the small quantities of the active materials that were available and by the lack of suitably sophisticated chromatographic and analytical techniques. It was not until 30 years later that Bergstrom and co-workers isolated the first prostaglandins in pure form and elucidated their structures.

Following this important breakthrough, research in Britain, Holland, Sweden and the USA has led to the discovery and structural elucidation of nine classes of prostaglandin.

Structures and nomenclature of prostaglandins

The nine classes of naturally occurring prostaglandins (PGs) that have been isolated to date are shown in *Figure 1.1.* The letters A–I were derived in the following way: the first successful purification of a prostaglandin in Sweden was accomplished by partition of the crude mixture between ether and phosphate buffer. Prostaglandin E was obtained from the ether phase (*e*ther), while prostaglandin F was isolated from the aqueous phase (*f*osfat). Treatment of prostaglandin E with *a*cid gave prostaglandin A while *b*ase treatment of the same substrate gave prostaglandin B. As other prostaglandins were discovered they were given the appropriate letters to fill the gaps and to extend the sequence.

The prostaglandins illustrated in *Figure 1.1* are given the subscript 2 to

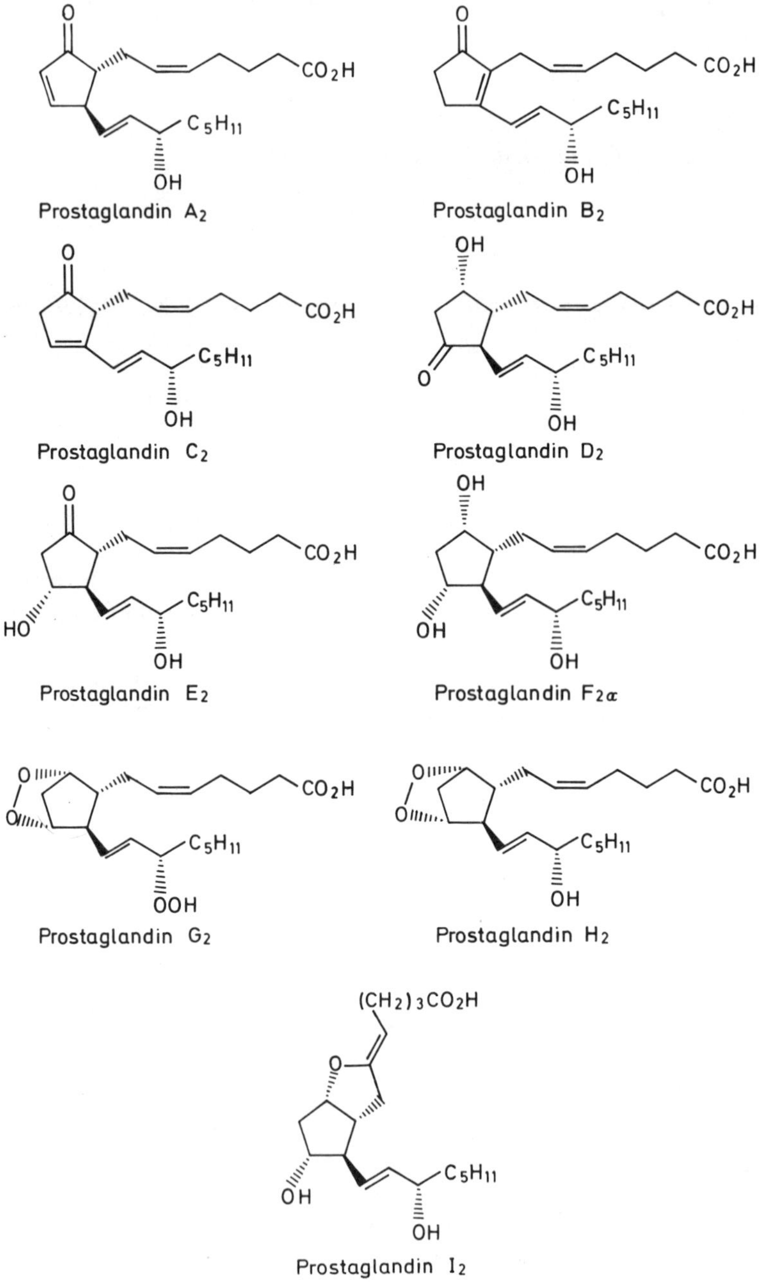

Prostaglandin A_2

Prostaglandin B_2

Prostaglandin C_2

Prostaglandin D_2

Prostaglandin E_2

Prostaglandin $F_{2\alpha}$

Prostaglandin G_2

Prostaglandin H_2

Prostaglandin I_2

Figure 1.1: The nine classes of naturally occurring prostaglandins isolated to date

signify the presence of two double bonds in the side chains. Analogous prostaglandins with one or three double bonds in the side chains are known also, as shown for prostaglandin E in *Figure 1.2*. The one exception is that prostaglandin I in the one series has not been found in nature. The numbering of the prostaglandins is conventional: the number 1 is given to the carbon atom of the principal group (*see* prostaglandin E_2 in *Figure 1.2*). Finally, the

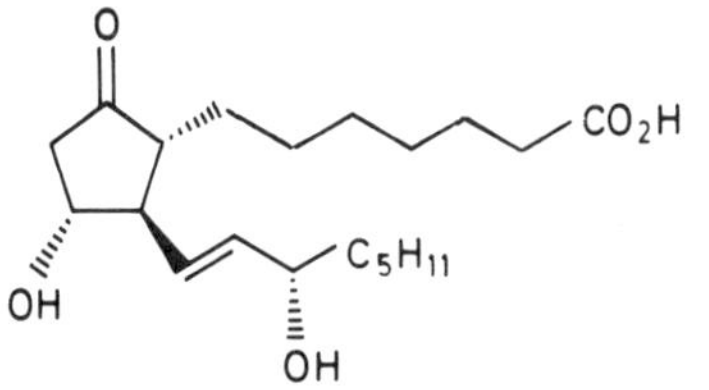

Prostaglandin E_1

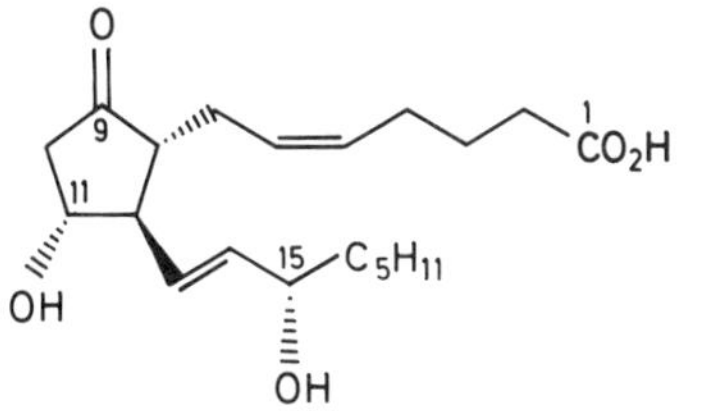

Prostaglandin E_2

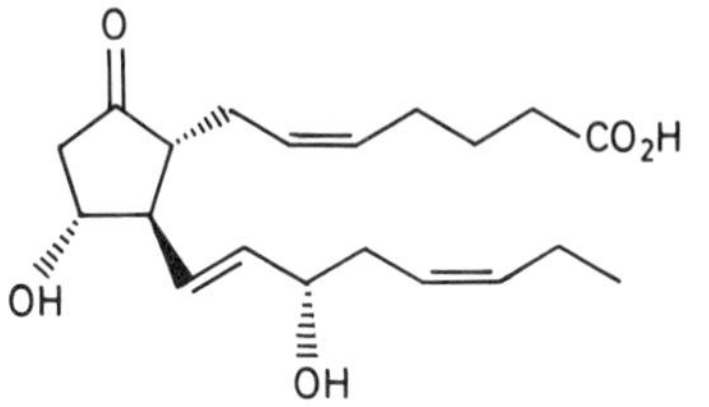

Prostaglandin E_3

Figure 1.2: The three series of prostaglandin E

subscript α — given to the F-family of prostaglandins — refers to the configuration of the hydroxyl group attached to C-9.

Substances closely related to prostaglandins have been isolated recently. These compounds have an oxacyclohexane ring in place of the cyclopentane ring of the prostaglandins and they have been dubbed thromboxanes because of their ability to induce aggregation of blood platelets and cause thrombus formation. Two classes of thromboxane have been isolated (*see Figure 1.3*).

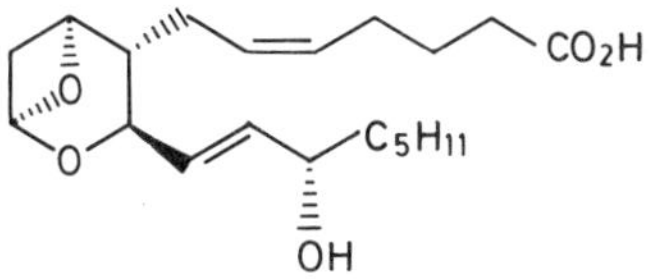

Thromboxane A_2

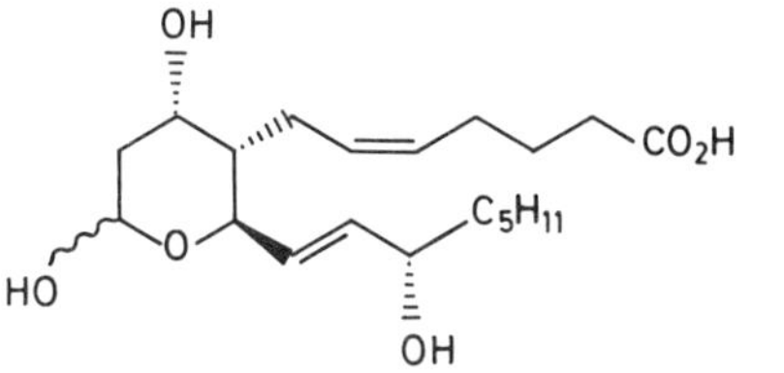

Thromboxane B_2

Figure 1.3: The structures of the thromboxanes

Thromboxane B_2 has been fully characterized, but the structure of thromboxane A_2 is based on mass spectral and chemical data only. Full spectroscopic analysis and chemical synthesis of this very unstable molecule have not been reported to date.

Synthetic analogues of the naturally occurring prostaglandins are called prostanoids.

Occurrence

Prostaglandins are widely distributed in mammalian tissues; the richest sources (*ca* 300 μg/g) of prostaglandins are the seminal fluids of man and sheep. Lower concentrations (*ca* 1 μg/g) are detectable in tissues from *inter alia* the uterus, lung, brain, eye, pancreas and kidney. Prostaglandin A_2-15-acetate has been obtained from the gorgonian *Plexaura homomalla*, a coral found in the Caribbean, while onions contain appreciable quantities of prostaglandin A_1. Prostaglandins E_2 and $F_{2\alpha}$ have been found in the red alga *Gracilaria lichenoides.*

Biosynthesis and metabolism

Prostaglandins are not stored in specialized cellular compartments, but are synthesized by the cell from long-chain polyunsaturated carboxylic acids in response to a stimulus. For instance, lungs synthesize and release relatively large quantities of prostaglandins in response to gentle stroking of the lung surface.

Oestrogens are well-known chemical stimulants for prostaglandin $F_{2\alpha}$ production within the uterus of species such as the guinea-pig and the sheep. Adrenaline stimulates prostanoid release from many tissues including the spleen, fat cells and the brain.

In general, prostaglandins are produced close to the site where they are to exert a biological effect and are then rapidly metabolized to less active materials. The major pathways of prostaglandin biosynthesis and the main metabolic breakdown pathways are illustrated in Chapter 2.

Potential clinical uses

Prostaglandins, thromboxanes and their analogues exhibit a wide range of biological activities. Some of these activities are briefly described below; a more detailed discussion is contained in Chapter 3.

Rheumatoid arthritis, a condition involving inflammation of a joint, is probably caused by over-production of prostaglandins in the diseased tissue. Prostaglandins E_1, E_2 and I_2 induce biological responses which together reproduce the classic picture of inflammation, namely redness, swelling and pain. The role of prostaglandins in modulating the production of pain is well established. Bradykinin and histamine are both potent pain-producers but their duration of action is shortlived. In the presence of prostaglandins the intensity and also the duration of the sensation is greatly enhanced. For example, responses to bradykinin and histamine after prostaglandin E_2 pretreatment lasted over half an hour, whereas without such pretreatment the duration was no more than a few minutes.

Corticosteroids and non-steroidal drugs such as aspirin and indomethacin reduce inflammation and alleviate pain by interfering with prostaglandin biosynthesis. Aspirin is a fatty acid cyclooxygenase inhibitor (*see* Chapter 2) and hence blocks the synthesis of all the prostaglandins. The steroid drugs act either by interfering with the mobilization of arachidonic acid (*see Figure 1.4*)

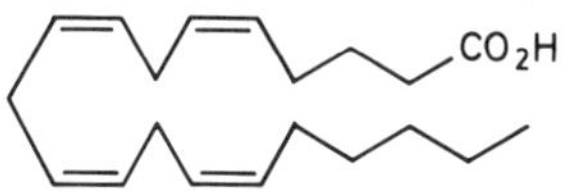

CO_2H

Figure 1.4: Arachidonic acid

from phospholipids (*see* Chapter 2) or by preventing the release (rather than the synthesis) of the prostaglandins. These two important classes of drugs found valuable and widespread therapeutic application long before their connection with the prostaglandin system was discovered.

A feverish condition in an animal can be induced by injection of prostaglandin E_2 into that region of the brain concerned with the regulation of body temperature. Further experiments have shown that the rise in body temperature and the concentration of endogenous prostaglandin E_2 in the appropriate region of the brain are directly related.

Prostaglandins E_2 and $F_{2\alpha}$ and some synthetic prostanoids have been used for the induction of labour and for the termination of pregnancy. Midterm abortions require higher doses of prostaglandins with the correspondingly higher incidence of side effects such as nausea, vomiting and diarrhoea. The routine monthly use of prostanoids to induce menstruation, whether or not conception has occurred, is one future approach to the control of human fertility. An alternative would be prostanoid administration as soon as the menstrual period has been missed.

In a related veterinary application, the prostanoids cloprostenol (Estrumate) and fluprostenol (Equimate) (*see Figure 1.5* and Chapter 8) are marketed by ICI to control the oestrus cycles of cattle and horses respectively as an aid to artificial insemination.

Prostaglandins of the E family inhibit gastric acid secretion in animals. On the other hand, the administration of both non-steroid and steroid anti-inflammatory drugs often causes serious adverse effects to the stomach. The established inhibition of prostaglandin production by these drugs may lead to an exposure of the stomach lining to damaging levels of gastric acid. Gastric ulceration may also result from under-production of prostaglandins; it has been observed that several synthetic prostanoids inhibit gastric acid secretion and promote the healing of peptic ulcers in human patients.

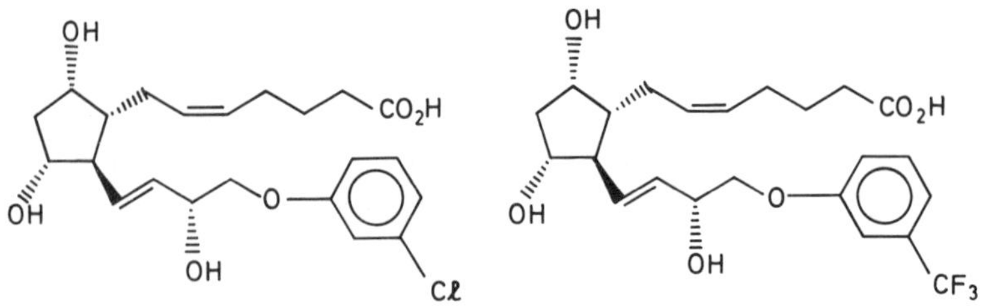

Estrumate Equimate

Figure 1.5: The structures of Estrumate and Equimate

Several prostaglandins inhibit the aggregation of human blood platelets: prostaglandin I_2 is particularly potent in this respect. In contrast, other prostaglandins, as well as thromboxane A_2, cause the aggregation of these platelets. Thromboxane A_2 is synthesized by the platelets themselves and leads to the spontaneous aggregation observed on contact with collagen, thrombin or a foreign body. Prostaglandin I_2 is produced by cells lining blood vessel walls (these cells contain the necessary synthetase enzyme), and leads to the lack of adherence of platelets to the healthy blood vessel wall. Diseased or damaged blood vessels probably produce lower concentrations of prostaglandin I_2; thromboxane production by the platelets in the vicinity will remain unaffected leading to platelet adhesion to the diseased vessel and ultimately to the formation of a potentially lethal thrombus. Redressing the prostaglandin I_2-thromboxane A_2 balance might prove to be a crucial aid to patients at risk from thrombosis or stroke.

Prostaglandins play a vital role in other systems. For example, they exert an effect on blood pressure and on bronchial smooth muscle, while their involvement in the central nervous system and with the onset of some forms of bone cancer has been mooted.

The relative concentrations of various prostaglandins at a particular site may be very important from a pharmacological standpoint; indeed, enzymes are known that interconvert prostaglandins of the D, E and F series.

In general, the over-production or the under-production of prostaglandin(s) at a particular site in the body can have a serious deleterious effect. Correction of this imbalance could be accomplished using a prostaglandin antagonist in the former case and either a natural prostaglandin or a synthetic prostaglandin agonist in the latter. The use of a natural prostaglandin in human chemotherapy is fraught with difficulties for two reasons: first, the rapid metabolic breakdown of the prostaglandin mitigates against the material reaching the desired site; secondly, a prostaglandin imbalance would almost certainly be created in other parts of the body leading to serious side effects due to the numerous biological activities of the molecule.

Under-production of a particular prostaglandin could be corrected by the administration of a suitable prostanoid (agonist) which binds specifically to the appropriate biological receptor and elicits the same response as that given by the natural material. Over-production of a particular prostaglandin could be moderated by the use of a prostanoid (antagonist) which binds strongly and specifically to the biological receptor at the correct site, but does not elicit the response caused by the natural prostaglandin. The success of such strategies relies on an intimate knowledge of the pharmacology of prostaglandins (*see* Chapter 3) and on appreciating the nature and identifying the number of prostaglandin receptors.

Thus, prostanoids are required that exhibit highly selective agonist or antagonist properties. The search for such molecules has generated a colossal amount of chemical research. The monocyclic prostaglandins have been prepared by stereocontrolled reactions involving polycyclic molecules (*see* Chapter 4) or by methods involving conjugate addition of nucleophiles to cyclopentenones (*see* Chapter 5). Prostaglandins G_2, H_2 and I_2 have been prepared by modification of prostaglandin $F_{2\alpha}$ (see Chapter 6): other prostaglandin interconversions are also described in Chapter 6. Thromboxanes have been prepared by methods closely related to those used in prostaglandin synthesis (*see* Chapter 7).

Successful routes to natural prostaglandins have been utilized to prepare prostanoids with modified side chains (*see* Chapter 8) and to provide prostaglandins with modified central-ring systems (*see* Chapter 9). These prostanoids often exhibit biological properties that are markedly different to the naturally-occurring compounds; these will be discussed in the relevant Chapters.

More recently, some thromboxane analogues have been prepared that are potent antagonists of the natural compounds (*see* Chapter 10).

CHAPTER 2

Biosynthesis and metabolism of prostaglandins and thromboxanes

Keith H. Gibson
Chemistry Department (II), ICI (Pharmaceuticals) Ltd., Alderley Park, Macclesfield, Cheshire

Introduction

In considering the biosynthesis of prostaglandins, this chapter will deal primarily with the detailed metabolism of arachidonic acid (1) leading to prostaglandins of the 2-series (e.g. $PGF_{2\alpha}$) in mammalian systems. So far as is known, the corresponding 1-series prostaglandins (e.g. $PGF_{1\alpha}$) derived from dihomo-γ-linolenic acid (2) and the 3-series (e.g. $PGF_{3\alpha}$) derived from 5,8,11,14,17-eicosapentaenoic acid (3) are biosynthesized by analogous reaction pathways where possible. Whilst prostaglandins do occur in non-mammalian systems, much less is known about their biosynthesis and function.

It is worth noting that the enzyme systems which produce prostaglandins are able to accept certain unnatural substrates and convert these into unnatural prostaglandins. For example, 2-methylarachidonic acid (4) can be fed to a prostaglandin-producing enzyme system which will convert it into the unnatural prostaglandin analogue 2-methyl-PGE_2 (5).

Although the biosynthesis of prostaglandins and related compounds is here considered in total, it cannot be stressed too strongly that the relative importance of the different prostaglandins varies enormously between different tissues and indeed also between the same types of tissue from different species. The availability of substrates, the different PG-synthesizing enzymes present (and active) together with the different rates of biosynthesis and metabolism can combine to make one particular prostaglandin predominate in any particular tissue. Thus PGD_2 seems to be the major product in rat brain, PGE_2 is found particularly in kidneys, PGI_2 predominates in blood vessel walls, and TXA_2 predominates in blood platelets. Furthermore, highly specific actions of different natural prostaglandins emphasize the different relative importance to different tissues: TXA_2 causes human blood platelets to aggregate, whereas PGI_2 causes them to disaggregate. PGI_2 also causes a specific relaxation of the bovine coronary artery.

Prostaglandins are not stored in mammalian cells, but are produced in response to stimulation. At the functional level, it appears that many prostaglandins are rapidly biosynthesized, exert their biological effect, and are rapidly metabolised, thereby functioning as autacoids or local hormones. However, some prostaglandins (possibly PGI_2) may have a half life of several minutes, which is sufficiently long to enable them to act over a wider range.

We now consider the individual steps of the biosynthetic pathways which start with the release of free arachidonic acid.

Prostaglandin biosynthesis

Availability of arachidonic acid

Arachidonic acid is stored in cells in the form of various esters. The phospholipids of membranes contain large amounts of arachidonic acid as the phosphatidyl esters of choline, inositol, serine and ethanolamine. It is also found in mono-, di-, and tri-glycerides and in cholesterol esters; it is possible that all these esters can function as sources of free arachidonic acid, depending on the particular cell type and the form of the stimulation which

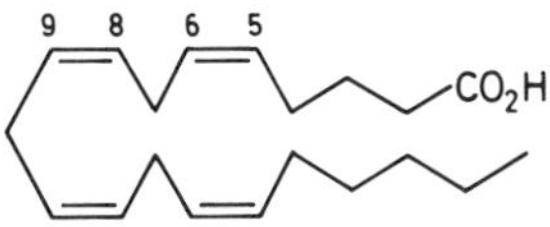

(1) 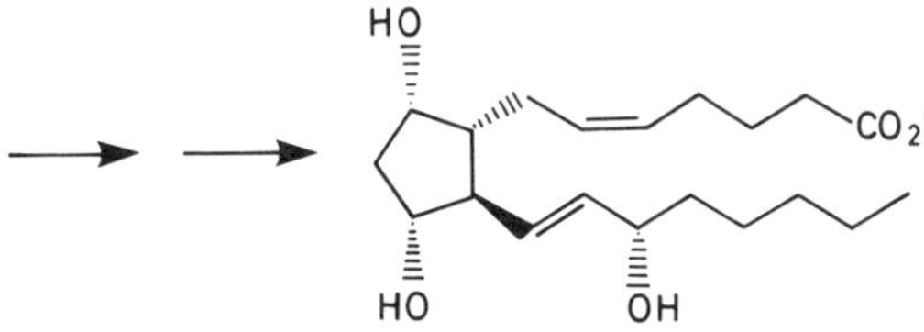 → → $PGF_{2\alpha}$

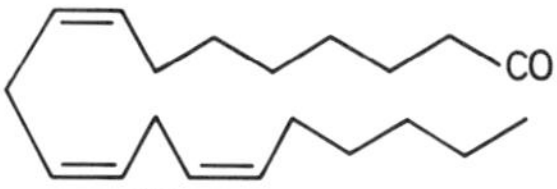

(2) 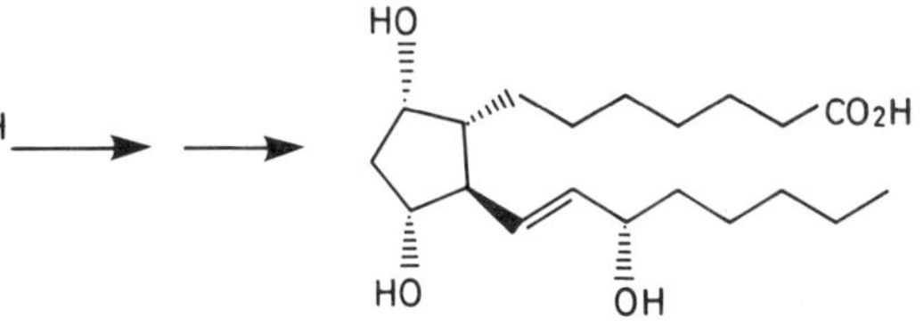 → → $PGF_{1\alpha}$

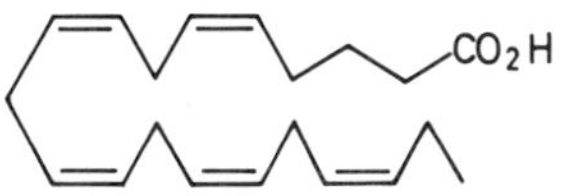

(3) 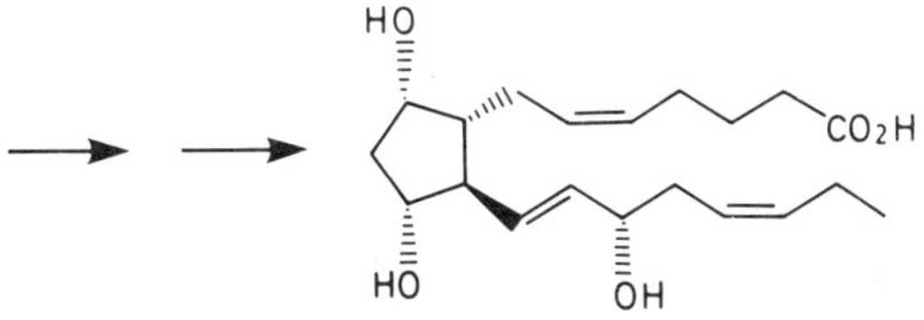 → → $PGF_{3\alpha}$

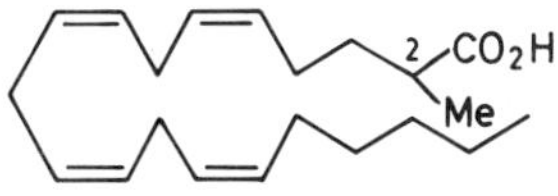

(4) 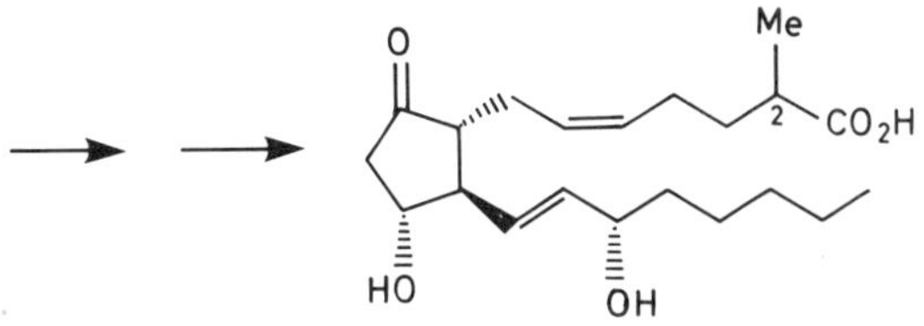 → → (5)

leads to the release of the arachidonic acid. Many different types of stimulation — physical (stretching, squeezing, vibration, electrical) and chemical (hormonal, immunological, ischaemia) — will lead to the release of free arachidonic acid.

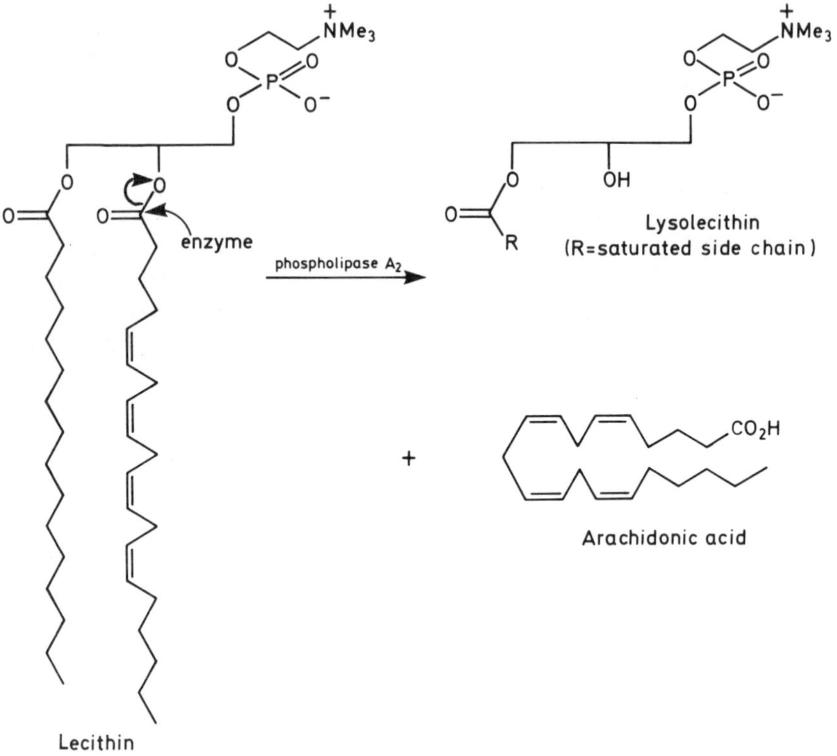

Figure 2.1: Release of arachidonic acid from lecithin

In many instances the phospholipid lecithin (phosphatidylcholine) appears to be the major source of released arachidonic acid. The release of arachidonic acid from the 2-position of lecithin is catalyzed by phospholipase A_2 enzymes, and this reaction has been studied very carefully (*see Figure 2.1*). The phospholipase A_2 enzymes are obtainable from several sources and are classified roughly into two types. Type I enzymes are bound to cellular membranes and their enzymic activity is related to the membrane stability. The Type II phospholipases are soluble enzymes found in many different mammalian cells. It is interesting that these mammalian enzymes are similar to the phospholipase A_2 enzymes found in the venoms of certain poisonous species such as bees, wasps, snakes, scorpions and Gila monsters. The mammalian Type II enzyme is produced as an inactive precursor — a prephospholipase — which is activated by the removal of a heptapeptide from the N-terminus of the prephospholipase. The phospholipase A_2 from bovine pancreas contains 123 amino acid units and has been obtained in good crystalline form, which has allowed X-ray crystallographic analysis to determine the three-dimensional structure[1].

The different phospholipase A_2 enzymes can exhibit quite different reactivities. Thus, while phospholipase A_2 from snake venom can attack lecithin within the tightly-packed structure of the native membrane, the mammalian phospholipase A_2 is unable to do this and can only release arachidonic acid from lecithin in the form of monomeric units or in loosely-packed micelles. Activating factors and inhibiting factors are also involved with the activity of the phospholipase A_2 enzymes. Endogenous small peptides and proteins can profoundly affect phospholipase A_2 activity; furthermore, these factors can themselves be influenced by drug administration. For example, in certain inflammatory conditions e.g. rheumatoid arthritis, the symptoms of inflammation are due, in part, to excessive production of prostaglandins which can act as inflammatory mediators. Corticosteroids such as dexamethasone have potent antiinflammatory activity and this activity correlates with the ability of the corticosteroid to prevent the release of the arachidonic acid which is the precursor of the prostaglandins. It now appears that the function of the corticosteroid is to stimulate the production of an endogenous peptide, which then acts as an inhibitor of phospholipase A_2 and thereby prevents the release of arachidonic acid.

Endoperoxide formation and isomerization (*see Figures 2.2 and 2.3*)

The enzyme systems responsible for the conversion of arachidonic acid into prostaglandins are often referred to as prostaglandin synthetase. However, these transformations involve several steps each having its own particular enzyme. The first step involves the interaction of one molecule of arachidonic acid with two *molecules* of oxygen in the enzyme system called prostaglandin cyclooxygenase to form the bicyclic endoperoxide PGG_2 which has a hydroperoxide function at C-15. *Figure 2.2* shows a proposed mechanism[2] for this reaction, but as yet there is no evidence for any detectable intermediates between arachidonic acid and PGG_2. However, chemical and electron spin resonance evidence indicate that the reaction does involve radicals. Studies with isotopically labelled arachidonic acid (tritium at C-13) and $^{18}O_2$ have shown that it is specifically the pro-*S* hydrogen at C-13 which is removed and that one *molecule* of oxygen provides both oxygen atoms at C-9 and C-11. Peroxidase activity results in the cleavage of the C-15 hydroperoxide to form the hydroxyl group present in PGH_2.

The cyclooxygenase activity requires haem as a cofactor and the peroxidase activity requires a hydrogen donor (e.g. tryptophan, serotonin, or adrenaline). The cyclooxygenase activity is only partially understood at present: it requires activation which may be some form of radical initiation; it is inhibited irreversibly by peroxides and reversibly by glutathione peroxidase; the enzyme action appears to catalyze the destruction of the enzyme itself; and the activity is inhibited by singlet oxygen scavengers.

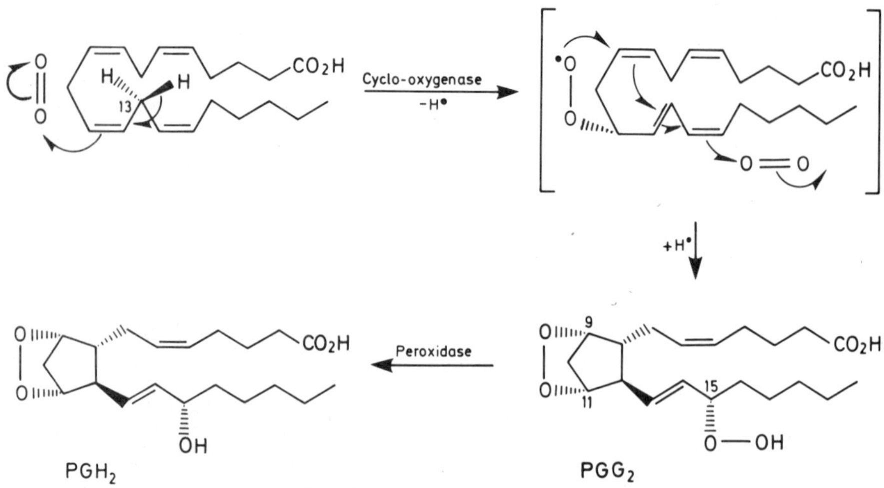

Figure 2.2: Biosynthesis of PGG_2 and PGH_2

The bicyclic endoperoxides PGG_2 and PGH_2 are the precursors of all the prostaglandins and thromboxanes and as such occupy the central role in the biosynthetic picture. They are also relevant in the pharmacological sense, because many important anti-inflammatory agents (e.g. aspirin (6) and indomethacin (7)) and antipyretic agents (e.g. paracetamol (8)) exert their action by inhibiting cyclooxygenase enzymes and thereby preventing the formation of the endoperoxides[3]. Experiments with radiolabelled aspirin have shown that aspirin irreversibly acetylates the cyclooxygenase enzyme.

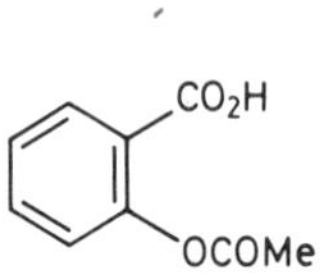

(6) 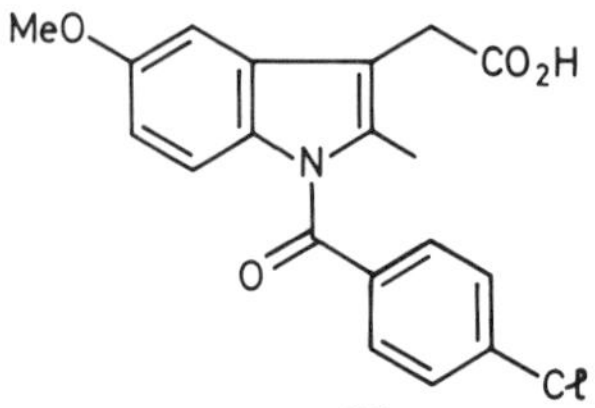 (7) 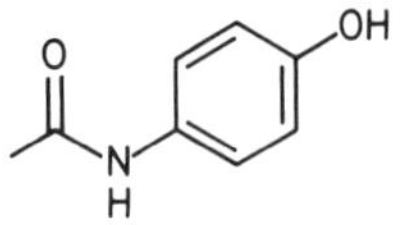 (8)

Two steps are required to convert PGG_2 into PGE_2: cleavage of the C-15 hydroperoxide to give a hydroxyl function by a peroxidase enzyme; and isomerization of the endoperoxide to the β-hydroxyketone by the PGE_2-isomerase enzyme. Probably these two steps can occur in either order and indeed the relative rates may depend on several factors. Mechanistically, the isomerization is simply the loss of a proton from C-9 with opening of the endoperoxide and protonation of the C-11 oxygen (*see Figure 2.3*). In analogous manner, the enzyme PGD_2-isomerase causes an alternative isomerization starting with loss of a proton from C-11 and thence leading to PGD_2 (*see Figure 2.3*). Reduction of the endoperoxide by endoperoxide reductase leads directly to $PGF_{2\alpha}$ which is also formed from PGE_2 by another important enzyme, prostaglandin-9-keto-reductase. Rat kidney contains a novel PG-9-hydroxydehydrogenase which oxidizes $PGF_{2\alpha}$ directly to PGE_2.

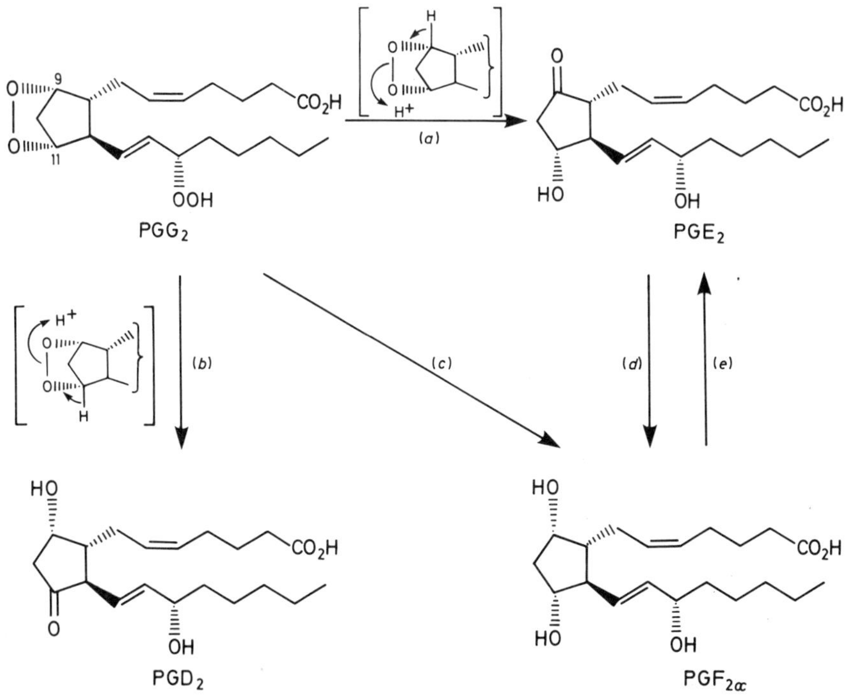

Enzymes: (*a*) PGE-isomerase and peroxidase; (*b*) PGD-isomerase and peroxidase; (*c*) Endoperoxide-reductase; (*d*) PG-9-keto-reductase; (*e*) PG-9-hydroxy-dehydrogenase

Figure 2.3: Enzymic interconversion of PGD_2, $PG\ E_2$, $PGF_{2\alpha}$ and PGG_2

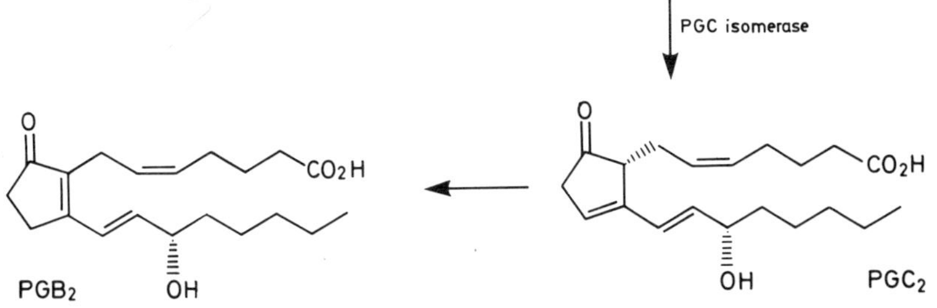

Figure 2.4: Interconversion of PGA_2, PGB_2, PGC_2 and PGE_2

PGE_2 transformations (*see Figure 2.4*)

PGE_2 readily dehydrates under acidic conditions to give PGA_2. Consequently, when PGA_2 is found in tissue samples it is not always clear whether this prostaglandin is an endogenous material or if it is an artefact derived from PGE_2 during the handling procedure. However, an enzyme — PGC isomerase — has been identified which can convert PGA_2 into PGC_2. PGC_2 readily isomerizes to PGB_2.

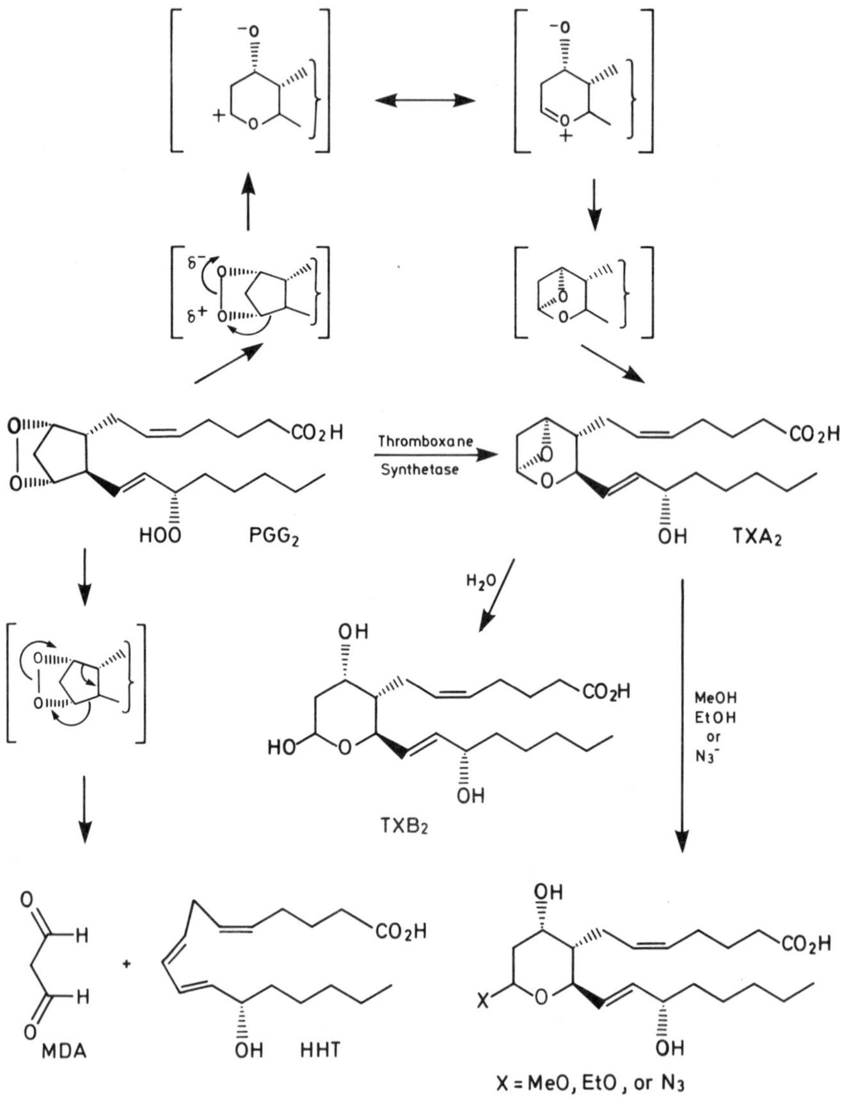

HOO PGG2
Thromboxane Synthetase
OH TXA2
H2O
MeOH EtOH or N3⁻
TXB2
MDA
OH HHT
X = MeO, EtO, or N3

Figure 2.5: Biosynthesis of the thromboxanes

Thromboxanes (*see Figure 2.5*)

The Swedish biochemists Samuelsson and Hamberg found that when washed human platelets (thrombocytes) were stimulated with thrombin, only very small amounts of PGE_2 and $PGF_{2\alpha}$ were formed[4]. However, they did discover the formation of a novel compound which they called thromboxane B_2 (TXB_2). They deduced that TXB_2 was formed from PGG_2 by rearrangement of the bicyclic endoperoxide to an intermediate thromboxane A_2 (TXA_2) with the unusual oxetane structure. This structure would be extremely labile and readily hydrolyze to form TXB_2. It was found that the putative intermediate could be trapped by added nucleophiles such as MeOH, EtOH or N_3^-. Evidence has now accumulated for the production of TXA_2 by many different tissues. The enzyme which converts endoperoxide into TXA_2 is called thromboxane synthetase and the mechanism is conceived as a polarization of the endoperoxide, followed by rearrangement as shown in *Figure 2.5*. The details of the mechanisms are not understood because the formation of TXA_2 seems to be accompanied by the formation of comparable amounts of malondialdehyde (MDA) and hydroxyheptadecatrienoic acid (HHT). These two compounds could be formed from endoperoxide PGG_2 by retro-Diels-Alder reaction, but the reason why it should accompany TXA_2 formation is not clear. TXA_2 is an extremely potent platelet aggregating agent, but it is a very labile compound and hydrolyzes to TXB_2 with a half-life of about 36 seconds in water at 37°C.

Prostacyclin (*see Figure 2.6*)

Microsomes of rabbit or pig aorta produce a labile but very potent inhibitor of platelet aggregation and this led Vane[5] and co-workers to identify in 1976 another novel prostanoid, prostacyclin (PGI_2; originally referred to as PGX). Subsequently, PGI_2 has been shown to occur in many different tissues. The formation of PGI_2 from endoperoxide by prostacyclin synthetase can be visualized as the polarization of the endoperoxide in the opposite sense to that required for TXA_2 formation. Participation of the 5,6-olefin could then lead to the formation of a secondary carbonium ion which, by loss of a proton from C-6, would give PGI_2. The enol-ether moiety of PGI_2 readily hydrolyzes under acidic conditions to give 6-keto-$PGF_{1\alpha}$.

In many situations, most notably in platelets, PGI_2 has pharmacological properties antagonistic to those of TXA_2. As both compounds are derived from the common endoperoxide precursor, the possibility exists that a subtle balance between the antagonistic properties of PGI_2 and TXA_2 maintains the physiologically normal state and that perturbations of this balance may be responsible for pathological conditions such as thrombosis, myocardial infarction and stroke.

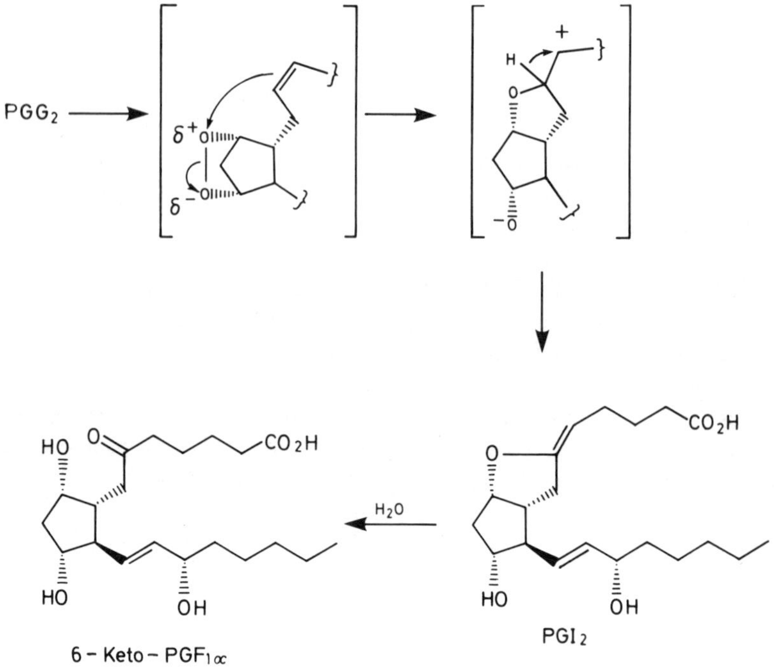

Figure 2.6. Biosynthesis of PGI_2.

Prostaglandin metabolism (*see Figure 2.7*)

As with the biosynthesis of prostaglandins, their metabolism and degradation occurs rapidly and to different extents in different tissues. Although a large number of metabolic pathways have been described, only the more important ones will be discussed here.

The primary deactivation step of $PGF_{2\alpha}$ is the oxidation of the 15-hydroxy function by the enzyme prostaglandin-15-dehydrogenase to give 15-keto-$PGF_{2\alpha}$. This enzymatic oxidation is particularly active in lung tissue, and greater than 95 per cent of $PGF_{2\alpha}$ present in the blood stream is deactivated by this mechanism on one passage through the lungs. Subsequently, the 13,14-double bond is reduced to give 13,14-dihydro-15-keto-$PGF_{2\alpha}$. The carboxylic acid side chain is then degraded by β-oxidation, which is the non-specific removal of two carbon atoms from the carboxylic acid terminus (β-oxidation can occur with all fatty acids). One stage of β-oxidation gives the dinor derivative (9), and removal of a second two-carbon fragment gives the tetranor derivative (10). Finally, the alkyl side chain is ω-hydroxylated to give (11) and then further oxidized to give the dicarboxylic acid (12), which is secreted as the major human urinary metabolite of $PGF_{2\alpha}$. PGE_2 is metabolized in an analogous manner to give (13).

The hydrolyses of TXA_2 to TXB_2 and of PGI_2 to 6-keto-$PGF_{1\alpha}$ occur

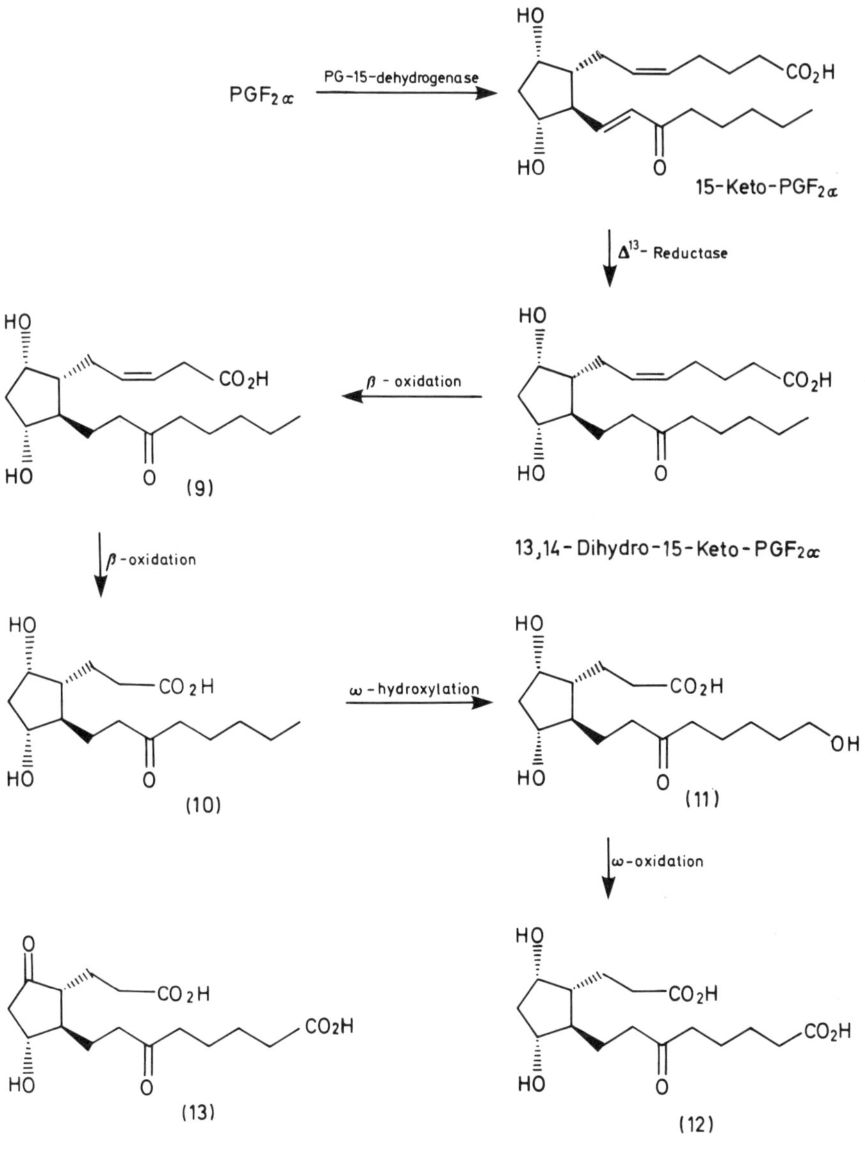

Figure 2.7: Metabolism of $PGF_{2\alpha}$

spontaneously, but may be enzyme assisted *in vivo*. In man, β-oxidation is the major metabolic pathway (*see Figure 2.8*) by which TXB_2 and 6-keto-$PGF_{1\alpha}$ are degraded and dinor-TXB_2 and dinor-6-keto-$PGF_{1\alpha}$ are the respective major urinary metabolites. 6-Keto-$PGF_{1\alpha}$ can also be converted into 6-keto-PGE_1 (which may be an important inhibitor of platelet aggregation) and to dinor-13,14-dihydro-6,15-diketo-$PGF_{1\alpha}$ (14) by analogous reactions to those of $PGF_{2\alpha}$ metabolism.

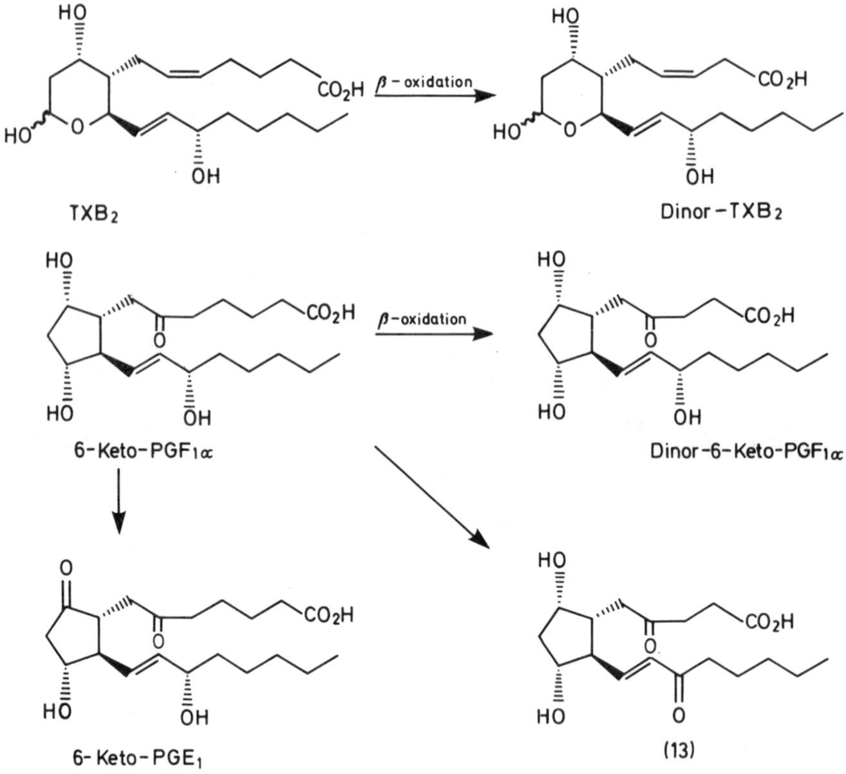

TXB2 → (β-oxidation) → Dinor-TXB2

6-Keto-PGF1α → (β-oxidation) → Dinor-6-Keto-PGF1α

6-Keto-PGE1

(13)

Figure 2.8: Metabolism of TXB_2 and 6-keto-$PGF_{1\alpha}$

References

1. B.W. DIJKSTRA, J. DRENTH, K.H. KALK and P.J. VANDERMAELEN, *J. molec. Biol.,* 1978, **124,** 53.
2. M. HAMBERG and B. SAMUELSSON, *J. Biol. Chem.,* 1967, **242,** 5336.
3. J.R. VANE, *Nature [New Biol.],* 1971, **231,** 232.
4. M. HAMBERG, J. SVENSSON, and B. SAMUELSSON, *Proc. natn. Acad. Sci. U.S.A.,* 1975, **72,** 2994.
5. S. MONCADA, R. GRYGLEWSKI, S. BUNTING and J.R. VANE, *Nature,* 1976, **263,** 663.

General references to further reading:

B. SAMUELSSON *et al., Ann. Rev. Biochem.,* 1975, **44,** 669.

K.C. NICOLAOU, G.P. GASIC and W.E. BARNETTE, *Angew. Chem. Int. Ed.,* 1978, **17,** 293.

K.C. NICOLAOU and J.B. SMITH, *Ann. Rep. Med. Chem.* 1979, **14,** 178.

CHAPTER 3

Pharmacology of natural prostaglandins and analogues

Ian Kennedy
Department of Pharmacology, Glaxo Group Research, Ware, Hertfordshire

Introduction

From the point of view of biologists, the two most striking features of the prostaglandins (PG) and thromboxanes (TX) are their widespread occurrence and broad spectrum of biological activity. These autacoids can be synthesized by almost every type of animal cell (the only well documented exception being the red blood cell), and almost every cell type can respond in some way to one or more of them. Furthermore, few substances have been subjected to more intensive and wide-ranging study in recent years and the literature on their biological actions is vast. For these reasons it is not possible to provide a comprehensive review of all aspects of the pharmacology of prostaglandins and thromboxanes. Therefore, this chapter concentrates on those aspects currently believed to be the most important, both physiologically and as potential targets for the medicinal chemist.

As described in Chapter 2, prostaglandins and thromboxanes are formed *in vivo* from eicosatrienoic acid, also known as dihomo-γ-linolenic acid (1-series compounds), eicosatetraenoic acid, more commonly known as arachidonic acid (2-series compounds), or eicosapentaenoic acid (3-series compounds). Under normal circumstances, arachidonic acid is the most abundant precursor in mammalian cells and there is little evidence that 1- and 3-series compounds are formed in significant amounts. Therefore, this review is mainly confined to the actions of 2-series compounds and the others will only be mentioned where their actions differ.

Mechanism of action of prostaglandins and thromboxanes

Prostaglandins and thromboxanes have such a wide range of biological actions that at first sight it might seem impossible to make useful generalizations about their mechanism of action. However, a number of lines of evidence suggest that they resemble other naturally occurring biologically active substances such as acetylcholine, histamine and the catecholamines, in that they produce their effects by interacting with specific receptors[1]. For example, prostaglandins are active at very low concentrations, sometimes as low as 10^{-11} mol/l. They also display a high degree of chemical specificity: that is small changes in chemical structure have profound effects on potency and there are marked differences in potency between different isomers of the same compound. These properties suggest the existence of highly specific recognition sites or receptors, which are probably situated in the cell membrane. Indeed, many studies have revealed the existence of specific prostaglandin-binding sites in the membranes of a number of cell types. However, in most cases it has yet to be established whether these are the receptors mediating the biological actions of prostaglandins or sites related to their transport or enzymatic inactivation.

Different prostaglandins often produce opposite effects on the same cell type. For example, TXA_2 causes blood platelets to aggregate, whereas PGI_2 inhibits platelet aggregation; some types of smooth muscle are contracted by $PGF_{2\alpha}$ but relaxed by PGE_2. Furthermore, different cell types respond to different prostaglandins. For example, platelets respond to TXA_2 and PGI_2, whereas PGE_2 and $PGF_{2\alpha}$ have little effect; in general the smooth muscle of the gastrointestinal tract responds to PGE_2 and $PGF_{2\alpha}$, while TXA_2 and PGI_2 are weakly active. These observations strongly suggest that more than one type of prostaglandin receptor exists. However, unlike histamine, acetylcholine, and the catecholamines, at present there is no generally agreed classification of the different types of prostaglandin receptors. The classification of prostaglandin receptors is of more than academic interest, since the numbers of different types and their distribution in different tissues will largely determine the degree of selectivity obtainable with synthetic compounds that mimic or block the effects of the natural compounds.

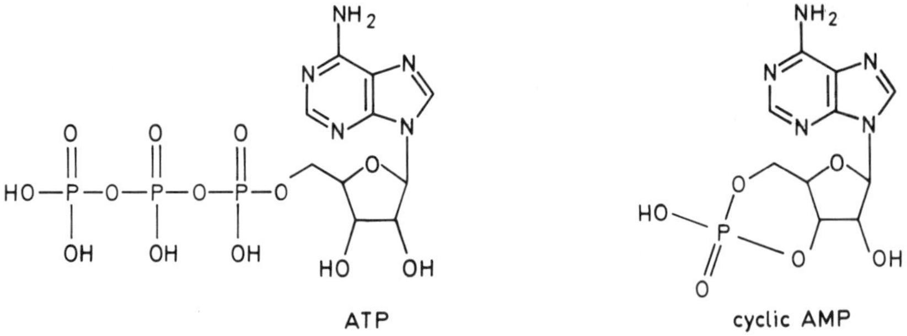

ATP

cyclic AMP

Figure 3.1

In many cases interaction of a hormone with its receptor stimulates the enzyme adenylate cyclase which catalyzes the formation of 3′,5′cyclic adenosine monophosphate (cyclic AMP) from adenosine triphosphate (ATP), which in turn acts as an intracellular second messenger to produce the response to the hormone (*see Figure 3.1*). For example, some of the actions of histamine and the catecholamines are mediated by stimulation of adenylate cyclase. Some of the actions of the E-series prostaglandins are also mediated in this way, as are the actions of PGI_2 and PGD_2 on platelets. The actions of

$PGF_{2\alpha}$ and TXA_2 do not seem to be mediated by stimulation of adenylate cyclase. The biochemical mechanisms involved in the actions of prostaglandins and thromboxanes not mediated by cyclic AMP are unknown; however, some might be mediated by increases in intracellular [Ca^{++}]. It has been suggested that in platelets the effects of TXA_2 might be mediated by an inhibition of adenylate cyclase, which produces a reduction in the intracellular concentration of cyclic AMP.

E-series prostaglandins

The E-series compounds, together with the F_α-series, were the first prostaglandins to be chemically characterized and synthesized and, until comparatively recently, were the most widely studied. In recent years, however, they have been overshadowed by the endoperoxides PGG_2 and PGH_2, the thromboxanes and PGI_2. Of all the prostaglandins, the E-series have probably the widest spectrum of actions, although it might be argued that this simply reflects the fact that they have been the most widely studied. They have potent actions on the cardiovascular, gastrointestinal, reproductive and respiratory systems. There is also strong evidence that they are mediators of inflammation, fever and certain types of pain.

Like all of the naturally occurring prostaglandins, the E-series compounds have a short duration of action *in vivo*, which can be measured in minutes following intravenous administration. In the case of the E-series and the F_α-series, the lung is a major site of inactivation; more than 90 per cent of a single dose of an E or F_α-series prostaglandin is inactivated in one passage through the pulmonary circulation[2]. This inactivation is accomplished by cellular uptake followed by enzymatic breakdown. This mechanism ensures that PGE_2 or $PGF_{2\alpha}$ released in peripheral tissues is inactivated before reaching the general circulation. It also has the practical consequence that PGE_2 or $PGF_{2\alpha}$ are less potent when administered intravenously than when administered intra-arterially.

E-series prostaglandins potently lower blood pressure in a variety of species including man. This hypotensive effect results from a direct relaxant action on vascular smooth muscle which produces vasodilatation involving most vascular beds[3]. There is reason to believe that this action is mediated by cyclic AMP. Cardiac output (the amount of blood pumped by the heart in unit time) is increased, however, this seems to be a reflex response to the vasodilatation and does not involve a direct action on the heart. PGE_2 and PGE_1 are approximately equipotent as vasodilators.

PGE_1 is a potent inhibitor of platelet aggregation (platelet aggregation and its physiological and pathological significance are described below), and this is believed to be a PGI_2-like effect. PGE_2 does not inhibit platelet aggregation, indeed in high concentrations it can potentiate aggregation.

Both PGE_1 and PGE_2 have potent actions on the kidney. They increase renal blood flow, urine formation and sodium and potassium excretion. The effects on urine formation and electrolyte excretion seem to result from direct action on the kidney, although increases in renal blood flow may also play a part.

Systemic administration of E-series prostaglandins to man produces nausea, vomiting, abdominal cramps and diarrhoea[4]. In experimental animals E-series prostaglandins are powerful diarrhoea-inducing agents. This seems to result from an increased movement of water and electrolytes into the lumen of the intestine, which is possibly mediated by cyclic AMP. Stimulation of gut propulsion resulting from an action on intestinal smooth muscle may also play a part. The effects of E-series prostaglandins on gastrointestinal smooth muscle vary with species and region of the intestine, but, in general, longitudinal smooth muscle is contracted and circular smooth muscle is relaxed. E-series prostaglandins are powerful inhibitors of gastric acid secretion. Since inhibitors of gastric acid secretion are used in the treatment of ulcers, there has been considerable interest in the possible use of prostaglandins in this area. There is some evidence that suggests that these compounds have an additional anti-ulcer action which is independent of their ability to inhibit acid secretion. The mechanism of this so called 'cytoprotective' action is unknown, but both modification of ion transport across the stomach wall and stimulation of mucus secretion have been suggested as possibilities.

E-series prostaglandins have powerful actions on the uterus. Non-pregnant human uterus *in vitro* is usually relaxed by E-series prostaglandins, whereas pregnant human uterus is contracted. In contrast, human uterus *in vivo*, whether pregnant or non-pregnant, is contracted by these compounds[5].

The reason for this difference is unknown. In man, monkeys and guinea-pigs, E-series prostaglandins are more potent uterine stimulants than are the F_{α}-series, whereas in rats the converse is true. PGE_2 has a luteolytic action (*see* below), but is less potent than $PGF_{2\alpha}$.

The most prominent symptom of asthma in man and anaphylaxis in guinea-pigs is bronchoconstriction, or narrowing of the airways, caused by contraction of airway smooth muscle. One approach to the treatment of these conditions is the use of substances, bronchodilators, which relax airway smooth muscle. Both PGE_1 and PGE_2 cause bronchodilatation in asthmatic subjects when administered as aerosols. This effect results from a direct relaxant action, which can be demonstrated on isolated airway smooth muscle from a variety of species including man. However, neither PGE_1 nor PGE_2 is suitable for the treatment of asthma, since when administered by aerosol both cause intense irritation and coughing and severe side effects preclude administration by any other route. Furthermore, in some asthmatic subjects these prostaglandins cause bronchoconstriction rather than bronchodilatation[6]. It is possible that some of this bronchoconstriction may be a reflex response to the irritant action, however, there is evidence that E-series prostaglandins have both contractile and relaxant actions on airway smooth muscle. Some synthetic PGE analogues may possess the bronchodilatory action without the bronchoconstrictory or irritant actions and might therefore be useful in the treatment of asthma.

There is an impressive body of evidence that implicates the prostaglandins as mediators of inflammation, fever and certain types of pain. The majority of work would suggest that E-series prostaglandins are the most important in this respect, although some recent studies also implicate PGI_2. The key finding that linked prostaglandins with inflammation, pain and fever was the discovery that the non-steroid anti-inflammatory (aspirin-like) drugs inhibit prostaglandin synthesis by blocking the cyclooxygenase enzyme. These drugs inhibit inflammation, relieve pain and reduce fever, and their potency is correlated with potency as inhibitors of prostaglandin synthesis. These findings have led to the view, now widely accepted, that non-steroid anti-inflammatory drugs exert their therapeutic effects by inhibiting prostaglandin synthesis[7].

Oedema (swelling) is one of the cardinal signs of inflammation and results from the passage of fluid out of small blood vessels and into the extracellular space consequent upon an increased permeability of the vessel wall. Prostaglandins E_1 and E_2 can increase vascular permeability, but they are much less effective than other inflammatory mediators such as histamine and bradykinin. However, both PGE_1 and PGE_2 markedly potentiate the increases in vascular permeability produced by substances such as histamine and bradykinin. This potentiation is believed to be a consequence of the vasodilator action of these prostaglandins, which increases blood flow to the inflamed area. Elimination of this potentiating effect is believed to be the basis of the anti-oedema action of aspirin-like drugs.

The involvement of prostaglandins in pain is also believed to be indirect[8]. Prostaglandins E_1 and E_2 can produce pain when administered on their own, but only at high concentrations which are unlikely to be achieved physiologically. However, both PGE_1 and PGE_2 (the former being more potent) can potentiate the pain-producing effects of other substances such as bradykinin. How this effect is produced is not known. Removal of this potentiation is believed to be the basis of the analgesic action of aspirin-like drugs. Since prostaglandins act by facilitating the pain-producing actions of other substances, this probably explains why these drugs are only effective against certain mild types of pain, particularly that associated with inflammation.

Prostaglandins E_1 and, to a lesser extent, E_2 are potent fever-inducing substances. Other prostaglandins lack this effect. Furthermore, fever-inducing agents, such as bacterial pyrogen, have been shown to cause prostaglandin release in the central nervous system, and both fever and the prostaglandin release can be blocked by aspirin-like drugs. It is therefore believed that inhibition of prostaglandin synthesis is the basis for the anti-pyretic action of aspirin-like drugs[9].

F_α-series prostaglandins

Like the E-series compounds, F_α-series prostaglandins were intensively studied during the early years of prostaglandin research, but have recently been neglected because of newer discoveries. Although they have a wide range of actions, most interest has centred on their effects on the female reproductive system, the lung and the gastrointestinal tract.

Prostaglandin $F_{2\alpha}$ powerfully contracts the smooth muscle of the uterus. As has already been described, it is more potent than PGE_2 in the rat, but in man the converse is true. A great deal of work has been done on the uterine stimulant action of prostaglandins, both from the point of view of their possible role in uterine function and as therapeutic agents for termination of pregnancy and induction of labour. However, the luteolytic action of prostaglandins has produced even greater interest. The corpus luteum is the body left behind when the ovum (egg) is expelled from the ovary. It produces the hormone progesterone which maintains the uterus in a quiescent state suitable for implantation and development of the egg. If pregnancy does not occur, then the corpus luteum regresses (luteolysis), progesterone secretion ceases, and menstruation occurs. It has been known for many years that in some species removal of the uterus prevents luteolysis, which suggests that the uterus produces a luteolytic hormone. There is now an overwhelming body of evidence that this luteolytic hormone is $PGF_{2\alpha}$[10]. The mechanism of action of $PGF_{2\alpha}$ has been a point of some controversy. Initial work showed that short-term incubation of isolated corpora lutea with $PGF_{2\alpha}$ stimulated progesterone secretion rather than inhibiting it. It was therefore suggested that luteolysis resulted from reduced ovarian blood flow caused by vasoconstriction. Another suggestion was that $PGF_{2\alpha}$ might inhibit release of luteotrophic hormones from the pituitary. However, subsequent studies demonstrated that $PGF_{2\alpha}$ does inhibit progesterone release from isolated corpora lutea upon prolonged incubation and it is now believed that this is the mechanism of action of $PGF_{2\alpha}$.

Demonstration of the luteolytic action of $PGF_{2\alpha}$ in species such as hamsters, rats, guinea-pigs and sheep raised the hope that such an effect might also occur in man. If $PGF_{2\alpha}$ had a luteolytic action in man, then it would be expected to be a post-coital contraceptive. Thus, inhibition of progesterone secretion from the corpus luteum immediately post-coitus would render the uterus unsuitable for development of the fertilized ovum, and pregnancy would be terminated. Indeed such a termination of early pregnancy is readily demonstrable in many laboratory animals. Unfortunately, in man and other primates, $PGF_{2\alpha}$ does not have a luteolytic action, and the early hopes that $PGF_{2\alpha}$ represented a novel type of contraceptive have not been realized.

The luteolytic action of $PGF_{2\alpha}$ has, nevertheless, found application in veterinary medicine. Administration of a luteolytic to a group of animals means that luteolysis and subsequent oestrus (heat) occur simultaneously and at a known time. It is therefore possible for a breeder to time mating and subsequent parturition. Species to which this technique has been applied include cattle, horses, sheep and pigs.

The lung was one of the first tissues found to synthesize $PGF_{2\alpha}$ and it was soon found that $PGF_{2\alpha}$ has a bronchoconstrictory action in the guinea-pig. In point of fact, $PGF_{2\alpha}$ is a rather weak bronchoconstrictor in the guinea-pig; it is much less potent than the prostaglandin endoperoxides and TXA_2. In the cat and dog, however, $PGF_{2\alpha}$ is a much more potent bronchoconstrictor. Findings such as these raised the possibility that $PGF_{2\alpha}$ might be a mediator of the bronchoconstriction which is such a prominent symptom of human asthma. Interest in this possibility was considerably heightened by the results of initial studies on the effects of $PGF_{2\alpha}$ on lung function in man. Asthmatics have hyperreactive airways and are more sensitive to the action of bronchoconstrictors than are non-asthmatics. An initial study found that whilst asthmatic subjects were 3–4 times more sensitive to the bronchoconstrictory action of aerosolized histamine than were normal subjects, they were some 8000 times more sensitive to aerosolized $PGF_{2\alpha}$. This dramatic result strongly supported the idea that $PGF_{2\alpha}$ might be a mediator of asthmatic bronchoconstriction. However, subsequent reports suggested that the hypersensitivity of asthmatics to $PGF_{2\alpha}$ was both less dramatic and more variable than that seen in the initial study[6], indeed in some subjects it is absent. Furthermore, studies on the effects of inhibitors of prostaglandin synthesis have not been encouraging. In the majority of asthmatic subjects, aspirin-like drugs are without effect. In a small proportion of asthmatics these drugs actually precipitate an asthmatic attack. This is possibly due to inhibition of the synthesis of a bronchodilator prostaglandin such as PGE_2. In a very small proportion of asthmatics, aspirin-like drugs have been claimed to have a beneficial effect, but in general the evidence available at present does not support the view that a bronchoconstrictor prostaglandin plays a major role in asthma[6].

Like PGE_2, $PGF_{2\alpha}$ has actions on the gastrointestinal tract. In contrast to PGE_2, which has both contractile and relaxant actions on gastrointestinal smooth muscle, $PGF_{2\alpha}$ in general causes only contraction. Furthermore, $PGF_{2\alpha}$ lacks the potent inhibitory action of the E-series compounds on gastric acid secretion and is less potent in causing fluid secretion into the intestine. In experimental animals, $PGF_{2\alpha}$ is less potent than PGE_2 or PGE_1 in producing diarrhoea.

$PGF_{2\alpha}$ lacks the potent vasodilatory actions of PGE_1 and PGE_2, it has a vasoconstrictory action in some vascular beds and increases in blood pressure have been reported in experimental animals. However, in general, the cardiovascular actions of $PGF_{2\alpha}$ are not prominent. $PGF_{2\alpha}$ has little or no effect on kidney function.

The prostaglandin endoperoxides

The existence of an endoperoxide intermediate in the synthesis of prostaglandins was originally postulated on theoretical grounds. Subsequently two such endoperoxides were isolated which differ only in that one has a hydroperoxy group at C-15 (PGG_2) whilst the other has a hydroxy group in this position (PGH_2)[11, 12]. PGG_2 and PGH_2 are chemically unstable, having half lives of about 5 minutes at 37°C in aqueous solution. They decompose into a mixture of varying proportions of PGD_2, PGE_2 and $PGF_{2\alpha}$. In addition they can be converted into other prostanoids by enzymes present in many tissues (*see* Chapter 2). Chemical instability makes these compounds difficult to work with and results are difficult to interpret since it is frequently not clear whether effects seen are mediated by endoperoxides themselves or by their products[13].

Despite these problems, there has been great interest in the biological actions of endoperoxides, particularly since they possess two actions that the classic stable prostaglandins lack. These are a powerful platelet aggregating action and a potent contractile action on some vascular smooth muscle preparations, perhaps the best known example being the rabbit aortic strip. These observations lead to the suggestion that the endoperoxides might not only serve as intermediates in the synthesis of prostaglandins but act as hormones in their own right. However, the subsequent discovery of TXA_2, which is even more potent in aggregating platelets and contracting vascular smooth muscle, suggested that the endoperoxides might be acting by initial conversion into this substance. Platelets readily convert endoperoxides into TXA_2 and it is therefore possible that their aggregating activity is due to conversion into endoperoxides. However, experiments with compounds that block the conversion of endoperoxides into TXA_2 have yielded contradictory results and at present it is unclear whether endoperoxides have to be converted into TXA_2 to aggregate platelets[13]. Blood vessels convert endoperoxides into PGI_2, and on those blood vessels that are not relaxed by PGI_2, such as rabbit aortic strip, the endoperoxides cause contraction which is presumably directly mediated. However, on those blood vessels which are relaxed by PGI_2, such as coronary arteries, endoperoxides cause relaxation which is mediated indirectly[14]. The direct contractile action of endoperoxides on vascular smooth muscle does not appear to be physiologically important since vasodilatation is the predominant response to endoperoxides in whole animals. It is possible that this vasodilatation is mediated by conversion into PGI_2.

Endoperoxides potently contract airway smooth muscle *in vitro* and cause bronchoconstriction *in vivo*[15]. They are more potent than $PGF_{2\alpha}$ but less potent than TXA_2. It is not clear whether the actions on airway smooth muscle are direct or indirect. Isolated intestinal smooth muscle is contracted by endoperoxides; in this case their potency is similar to or slightly less than that of PGE_2 and $PGF_{2\alpha}$[15]. Again it is unclear whether these effects are mediated directly or indirectly.

PGH_1 and PGH_3 can be formed from eicosatrienoic acid and eicosapentaenoic acid, respectively. The 1- and 3-series endoperoxides resemble the 2-series compounds in contracting isolated blood vessels such as rabbit aorta, but are somewhat less active[16]. PGH_3 relaxes those blood vessels, such as coronary arteries, that are relaxed by PGH_2, presumably by conversion into PGI_3. However, PGH_1 contracts these blood vessels, presumably because it cannot be converted into PGI_1. In contrast to PGH_2, neither PGH_1 nor PGH_3 cause platelet aggregation; indeed both can inhibit

PGH_2-induced platelet aggregation. In the case of PGH_3 this inhibition is probably mediated by breakdown to PGD_3[17].

D-series prostaglandins

PGD_2 was originally discovered during the isolation of the prostaglandin endoperoxides. Initial studies suggested that it had little biological activity and for some time D-series prostaglandins were neglected by pharmacologists. Subsequently, however, it has been found that PGD_2 has a distinct and interesting profile of biological activity of its own. Nevertheless, D-series prostaglandins have not been studied as extensively as the E- and Fα-series compounds, and many gaps in their pharmacology remain to be filled. The majority of the work carried out to date has been on the cardiovascular and respiratory system.

PGD_2 is a potent vasopressor agent in the anaesthetized sheep, being 70 times more potent than $PGF_{2\alpha}$[18]. PGD_2 does not appear to have this action in other species examined although vasoconstrictor actions in some vascular beds, for example the mesenteric vasculature of the dog, have been reported. On the other hand, vasodilatation has been observed in other vascular beds, for example the renal vascular bed of the dog. The renal vasodilatory action of PGD_2 is shared by PGE_2 and PGI_2. These latter two compounds also increase urine formation and electrolyte excretion. The cardiovascular actions of PGD_2 in man *in vivo* do not appear to have been described.

Perhaps the most interesting discovery has been that PGD_2 potently inhibits platelet aggregation, and is more active than PGE_1, but less active than PGI_2. Subsequently it was found that the anti-aggregatory action of PGD_2 is species dependent. PGD_2 inhibits the aggregation of human, sheep and horse platelets, but has no effect on rat or rabbit platelets. PGE_1 and PGI_2 inhibit platelet aggregation in all species studied and it seems likely that PGD_2 acts at a different receptor than do PGE_1 and PGI_2. This receptor is present on the platelets of man, horses and sheep, but not those of rats or rabbits. It is interesting to note that those species whose platelets are sensitive to PGD_2 are those whose plasma is most active in converting endoperoxides into PGD_2. It is therefore possible that PGD_2 may have a physiological role in the control of platelet aggregation in these species[19].

PGD_2 has been found to contract airway smooth muscle of the guinea-pig *in vitro* and is reported to be more active than $PGF_{2\alpha}$ and of similar potency to PGH_2[15]. Similarly, PGD_2 causes bronchoconstriction in the anaesthetized guinea-pig and dog. Its actions on human airways have not been described.

Little work has been carried out on the effects of PGD_2 on the gastro-intestinal system. PGD_2 generally contracts intestinal smooth muscle, but is less potent than PGE_2 and $PGF_{2\alpha}$. PGD_2 is a very weak inhibitor of gastric acid secretion and does not cause diarrhoea.

As has already been described, PGH_3 inhibits platelet aggregation by conversion into PGD_3. Although the pharmacology of PGD_3 has not been described in detail, it has been claimed that it has little effect on vascular and intestinal smooth muscle and that therefore PGD_3 might be a superior therapeutic agent to PGI_2[17].

Thromboxanes

Piper and Vane[20] demonstrated the release of a previously unknown substance, which they termed rabbit aorta contracting substance or RCS, from guinea-pig isolated perfused lungs. This substance potently contracts rabbit isolated aortic strips and many other isolated vascular smooth muscle preparations. It is highly unstable and has a half life of less than 2 minutes at 37°C. Release of RCS can be caused by a variety of stimuli including antigen challenge of sensitized lungs, mechanical trauma, and administration of arachidonic acid and some hormones such as bradykinin. RCS release can be blocked by aspirin-like drugs. These observations suggested that RCS is a cyclooxygenase product. The discovery that the unstable endoperoxides contract rabbit aorta raised the possibility that RCS was an endoperoxide. However, quantitative studies showed that the half life of RCS (less than 2 minutes) was shorter than that of the endoperoxides (about 5 minutes). Furthermore, the amounts of endoperoxide present in lung effluent were insufficient to account for the rabbit aorta contracting activity.

It was found that RCS was released by aggregating platelets and these studies revealed its structure. It was previously shown that the major stable cyclooxygenase product in platelets was a hemiacetal derivative initially called PHD and now termed TXB_2. A highly unstable intermediate in the conversion of PGH_2 into TXB_2 was isolated and termed TXA_2[21]. TXA_2 has a half life of about 30 seconds at 37°C and is more active than PGH_2 in contracting rabbit aorta. TXA_2 is the major constituent of RCS.

In addition to its action on vascular smooth muscle, TXA_2 aggregates platelets and is again more potent than PGG_2 and PGH_2. As has already been described, there is controversy as to whether the endoperoxides have to be converted into TXA_2 to produce platelet aggregation. However, although this question has yet to be finally resolved, under normal circumstances *in vivo* it seems plausible to assume that endoperoxides cause platelet aggregation through conversion into the more potent TXA_2[13]. Because of its extreme instability and difficulty of preparation, studies on the actions of TXA_2 in whole animals are very limited. It has been found to cause vasoconstriction in some vascular beds, for example the coronary and mesenteric beds.

TXA_2 potently contracts guinea-pig and human airway smooth muscle *in vitro*. Bronchoconstriction following intravenous administration to the anaesthetized guinea-pig has also been demonstrated[22]. It might therefore be anticipated that TXA_2 would be a potent bronchoconstrictor in man; however, this has not yet been studied.

As already described, guinea-pig lung readily produces TXA_2, and it is possible that TXA_2 mediates part of the bronchoconstriction of anaphylaxis in this species. Although human airways respond to TXA_2, it appears that human lung does not produce this substance. Thus on present evidence it is difficult to see how TXA_2 could contribute to asthmatic bronchoconstriction. Nevertheless, increased blood concentrations of the breakdown product of TXA_2, TXB_2, have been reported during an asthmatic attack.

At present little is known about the actions of TXA_2 on systems other than the cardiovascular and respiratory. In general TXA_2 has weak contractile actions relative to PGE_2 and $PGF_{2\alpha}$ on gastrointestinal smooth muscle. Its actions on gastric and intestinal secretion are unknown. Very little work has been done on the effects of TXA_2 on the reproductive system, although it has been reported to contract human and guinea-pig, but not rat, uterine smooth muscle *in vitro*.

The enzyme thromboxane synthetase converts PGH_1 into TXA_1 only to a very limited extent, and since chemical synthesis of thromboxanes A has not been achieved, the biological activity of TXA_1 is unknown. TXA_3 can be formed from PGH_3 and has been found to contract the isolated rabbit aorta, although it is less active than TXA_2. In contrast, TXA_3 does not aggregate platelets, suggesting that the thromboxane receptors in platelets and rabbit aorta may be different[16]. The stable breakdown product of TXA_2, TXB_2, has been reported to have weak contractile activity on some isolated smooth muscle preparations. However, TXB_2 is many times less potent than TXA_2, and it is most unlikely that these actions are of any physiological significance.

I-series prostaglandins

The discovery of PGI_2 arose from experiments designed to investigate the possibility that blood vessels might produce TXA_2 which could act synergistically with that produced by platelets. When blood vessels were incubated with endoperoxides, no TXA_2 was formed. However, a substance was formed which is in many ways the biological mirror image of TXA_2. This substance, which was termed PGX prior to the elucidation of its chemical structure, was found to relax certain isolated vascular smooth muscle preparations and also to be a very potent inhibitor of platelet aggregation.

Following the elucidation of its chemical structure, PGX was designated PGI_2 and given the trivial name prostacyclin. Prostacyclin is chemically unstable, more so in acid than alkali, having a half life of about 5 minutes at 37°C and physiological pH. It decomposes to 6-keto-$PGF_{1\alpha}$ which has little or no biological activity. Prostacyclin is the most potent known naturally occurring inhibitor of platelet aggregation, being up to 40 times more potent than PGE_1 and PGD_2 *in vitro*[13]. In whole animals, low concentrations of prostacyclin applied locally can inhibit platelet aggregation caused by adenosine diphosphate (ADP) and, when administered systemically, prevent platelet aggregation on the wall of an artery damaged by electrical stimulation. It can also increase bleeding time, probably by virtue of its anti-platelet action, although vasodilatation may also play a part. Not only does prostacyclin inhibit platelet aggregation, but it can also disaggregate already aggregated platelets.

As already noted, prostacyclin relaxes some isolated vascular smooth muscle preparations. It is also a potent vasodilator in whole animals. Unlike the E-series prostaglandins, prostacyclin is not inactivated by the lungs and its potency relative to the E-series compounds varies with route of administration. When both compounds are administered intravenously, prostacyclin is more potent than PGE_2, but when administered intra-arterially, so as to bypass the lungs, the potency of prostacyclin is similar to or less than that of PGE_2. The vasodilatory action of prostacyclin has been demonstrated in a range of vascular beds, including the coronary, renal and mesenteric. In contrast to PGE_2, which stimulates the heart (*see* above) in anaesthetized dogs, prostacyclin decreases heart rate. These cardiac effects also appears to be mediated by a reflex mechanism. However, in man, intravenously administered prostacyclin produces vasodilatation accompanied by an increase in heart rate.

The vasodilator actions of prostaglandins contribute to their pro-inflammatory actions (*see* above). The finding that 6-keto-$PGF_{1\alpha}$ is present in inflammatory exudates, together with the potent vasodilator actions of prostacyclin, suggests that prostacyclin may be a mediator of inflammation[13]. Prostacyclin also shares the ability of E-series prostaglandins to potentiate the effects of pain-producing substances (*see* above) and could therefore be involved in certain types of aspirin-sensitive pain.

Prostacyclin has potent actions on the kidney, causing vasodilatation, increased urine formation and electrolyte excretion, and since it can be formed in the kidney it may be an important renal hormone. In addition to those effects, which are shared by E-series prostaglandins, prostacyclin powerfully stimulates the release of renin from the kidney. Renin is an enzyme which catalyzes the formation of the vasoconstrictor peptide hormone angiotensin which probably plays a role in the regulation of the cardiovascular system.

Like PGE_1 and PGE_2, prostacyclin is a powerful inhibitor of gastric acid secretion. It also dilates the blood supply of the stomach and may have a physiological function since it is the major cyclooxygenase product of the gastric mucosa of several species. In contrast to the E-series prostaglandins, prostacyclin does not cause diarrhoea. It is only weakly active in contracting gastrointestinal smooth muscle and does not cause fluid secretion into the intestine. Indeed in experimental animals, prostacyclin has been found to inhibit the effects of other prostaglandins on fluid secretion.

Although prostacyclin shares the powerful relaxant action of PGE_1 and PGE_2 on vascular smooth muscle, it lacks their potent effects on airway smooth muscle and is not a potent bronchodilator. Prostacyclin is the major cyclooxygenase product in rat uterus. The function of prostacyclin in this species is uncertain, although it has been speculated that it might be involved in the regulation of uterine blood flow.

PGI_1 cannot be formed from PGH_1 by the enzyme prostacyclin synthetase. However, this compound has been synthesized chemically. It is chemically stable and shares the actions of PGI_2 on platelets and vascular smooth muscle although it is much weaker. PGI_1 also inhibits gastric acid secretion. PGI_3 can be formed enzymatically from PGH_3, it inhibits platelet aggregation and relaxes vascular smooth muscle and is of similar potency to PGI_2.

Thromboxane, prostacyclin and thrombosis

Arterial thrombosis is believed to be one of the major causes of heart attacks and strokes. Furthermore, platelet aggregation is believed to be the initiating event in arterial thrombosis. For these reasons the discovery of the potent actions of thromboxane and prostacyclin on platelets has generated enormous interest, since manipulation of the thromboxane-prostacyclin system offers several possible approaches to the prevention of thrombosis.

When blood platelets are exposed to a foreign surface or a damaged blood vessel wall, they clump together (aggregate) and release a number of substances, notably TXA_2, 5-hydroxytryptamine and ADP, which are vasoactive and promote further aggregation. When a small blood vessel is cut, a platelet aggregate, or haemostatic plug, forms at the site of the hole and is the foundation for a blood clot. Formation of the haemostatic plug is the physiological function of platelets; however, if the inner wall of the blood vessel is diseased or damaged then thrombus formation may occur. This thrombus may grow until it occludes the blood vessel, or it may break away and occlude a smaller blood vessel. If a coronary artery is occluded then myocardial infarction results; if a cerebral artery is occluded then a stroke results.

The production of prostacyclin by blood vessels and thromboxane by platelets represents an elegant mechanism for the control of platelet aggregation[13]. Platelets do not aggregate when exposed to the normal blood vessel wall and it is likely that this can be attributed largely, possibly entirely, to prostacyclin production. Prostacyclin production is confined to the innermost layer of the blood vessel wall, the vascular endothelium, and consequently removal of or damage to this layer will prevent prostacyclin production and allow platelets to aggregate.

Initial work suggested that, although blood vessels could generate prostacyclin from PGH_2, they could not do so from arachidonic acid. This led to the suggestion that aggregating platelets 'feed' endoperoxides to the vascular endothelium which converts them into prostacyclin. Subsequently it was found that blood vessels can synthesize prostacyclin from arachidonic acid, and at present there is controversy as to whether platelet-drived endoperoxides are used for prostacyclin synthesis. Prostacyclin is not inactivated on passage through the lungs, and indeed it has been shown that the lungs of experimental animals can release prostacyclin. This has led to the suggestion that prostacyclin released from the lungs acts as a circulating antiaggregatory agent, reinforcing the action of locally synthesized prostacyclin[23].

Platelets will aggregate when exposed to areas where the vascular endothelium is absent or damaged and hence where prostacyclin production is absent or impaired. TXA_2 is only one of a number of endogenous aggregatory substances, and its relative importance in platelet aggregation *in vivo* is at present unclear. However, low doses of aspirin that selectively inhibit platelet cyclooxygenase (*see* below) have been shown to prolong bleeding time, which suggests a role for thromboxane in the formation of the haemostatic plug.

There are a number of ways in which the thromboxane-prostacyclin system might be manipulated to prevent thrombosis.

1. The use of drugs, which block the cyclooxygenase enzyme, to prevent endoperoxide and TXA_2 formation.
2. The use of drugs which block the conversion of PGH_2 to TXA_2 (thromboxane synthetase inhibitors) or block the actions of TXA_2 (thromboxane antagonists).
3. The use of stable analogues of prostacyclin.
4. Manipulation of cellular fatty acids.

Prior to the discovery of prostacyclin, the use of cyclooxygenase inhibitors seemed a rational approach to the prevention of thrombosis. However, the discovery of prostacyclin made this a less attractive approach, since these drugs would be expected to block the formation not only of the prothrombotic thromboxane, but also of the antithrombotic prostacyclin. Nevertheless, it has recently been found that low doses of aspirin selectively block the platelet cyclooxygenase enzyme but have little effect on the vascular enzyme. Higher doses block both enzymes. It has therefore been suggested that low doses of aspirin should be more effective in the prevention of thrombosis than high doses[24]. It has further been suggested that the equivocal results obtained in clinical trials of aspirin in the prevention of thrombosis may be attributable to the use of doses that are too high.

There has been considerable interest in the possible use of inhibitors of the conversion of PGH_2 into TXA_2 as antithrombotics. Imidazole (1) was the first selective thromboxane synthetase inhibitor to be described; it is a comparatively weak compound but a number of more potent analogues have recently been discovered, for example (2). The value of thromboxane synthetase inhibitors as antithrombotics is at present unknown, but has been the subject of much debate. It has been suggested that inhibition of thromboxane synthetase could not only prevent TXA_2 formation, but that the resulting surplus endoperoxides might be converted into prostacyclin by the blood vessel wall. Evidence that this can occur *in vitro* has been obtained, although it is not known if this diversion occurs *in vivo*[13]. On the other hand the unconverted endoperoxides might cause platelet aggregation themselves. A compound which blocks platelet thromboxane receptors might also be valuable, although diversion of endoperoxide metabolism to prostacyclin could not occur. A few such compounds have been described, for example (3), but their value as antithrombotics is at present unknown.

A stable orally-active analogue of prostacyclin might also be a valuable

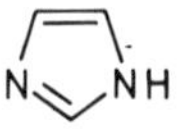

(1) 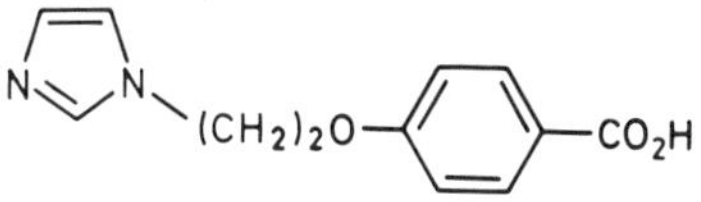 (2)

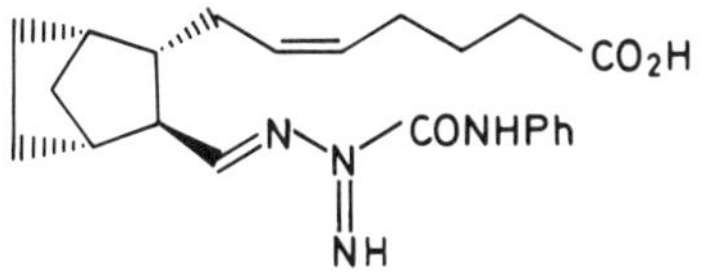

(3)

antithrombotic. Prostacyclin itself is unsuitable because of its instability and short duration of action *in vivo*. However, prostacyclin has been successfully used in experimental animals and man to prevent platelet aggregation and reduce the requirement for anticoagulants in extracorporeal circulation, for example during renal dialysis, cardiopulmonary bypass and charcoal haemoperfusion[25]. In these situations the short duration of action may be advantageous. Administration of prostacyclin to man at doses which inhibit platelet aggregation is accompanied by vasodilatation and hypotension. These effects would probably be undesirable in an antithrombotic; a prostacyclin analogue which inhibited platelet aggregation without causing vasodilatation would be preferable. A prostacyclin analogue would have the theoretical advantage over a thromboxane synthetase inhibitor or antagonist that it would be effective against aggregatory agents such as ADP whose action is independent of TXA_2.

Platelets cannot form TXA_1 and PGH_1 does not aggregate platelets; similarly TXA_3, though it can be formed, lacks aggregatory activity. There has been some interest in exploiting these findings for the prevention of thrombosis. It was suggested that addition of the precursor of the 1-series compounds, dihomo-γ-linolenic acid, to the diet might have an antithrombotic effect. However, the vascular endothelium cannot form PGI_1, thus formation of both pro- and antithrombotic prostanoids could be reduced, and results obtained with dihomo-γ-linolenic acid in experimental animals have not been encouraging. Use of the precursor of the 3-series compounds, eicosapentaenoic acid, might be more rational, since PGI_3 can be formed and is antiaggregatory. Indeed it has been suggested that the low incidence of myocardial infarction in Eskimos and their increased tendency to bleed could be due to the high eicosapentaenoic acid and low arachidonic acid content of their diet[26] (eicosapentaenoic acid is a major constituent of the fatty acids of marine animals).

A-, B- and C-series prostaglandins

Although most workers now consider it unlikely that these prostaglandins occur naturally in mammals, a certain amount of work on their pharmacology has been carried out. Early studies demonstrated that in whole animals PGA_1 and PGA_2 were vasodilators and inhibitors of gastric acid secretion of comparable potency to PGE_1 and PGE_2 when administered intravenously. However, the A-series compounds were found to be very weakly active relative to the E-series on isolated smooth muscle preparations. These findings raised the hope that A-series compounds might show greater selectivity of action than E-series and therefore be of greater potential value as therapeutic agents. However, this selectivity is probably illusory. Unlike the E-series compounds, PGA_1 and PGA_2 are not inactivated by passage through the lungs and when administered intra-arterially the A-series compounds are weakly active relative to the E-series.

Prostaglandins of the B-series are in general even less active than those of the A-series. It has been reported that PGB_1 and PGB_2 are more potent than PGE_2 and $PGF_{2\alpha}$ in contracting isolated blood vessels. However, PGE_2 and $PGF_{2\alpha}$ are extremely weakly active on these preparations and the potency of PGB_1 and PGB_2 is still very much less than that of the prostaglandin endoperoxides and TXA_2.

PGC_2 is chemically unstable, and very little work on its biological activity has been described. PGC_2 is a vasodilator, being more potent than PGA_2 but less potent than PGE_2. As has already been stated, the plasma of some species contains an enzyme which converts PGA_2 into PGC_2, and it is possible that in these species conversion into PGC_2 accounts for some of the vasodilatation produced by PGA_2.

Therapeutic applications of prostaglandins

The extremely wide range of biological actions of prostaglandins and thromboxanes has raised hopes that these substances or analogues of them might find application in the treatment of a variety of disorders. The prevention of thrombosis, currently the most exciting possibility, has already been discussed, as have the veterinary applications of luteolytic prostaglandins.

To date the most successful therapeutic applications of prostaglandins and prostaglandin analogues has been in the field of obstetrics and gynaecology. PGE_2, $PGF_{2\alpha}$ and synthetic analogues of them have been used successfully both for induction of labour and for the termination of unwanted pregnancy. Originally intravenous infusions were used, but at parturition oral or intra-uterine administration is often effective and more acceptable. For these reasons the intravenous route has largely been superseded. As has already been described, hopes that $PGF_{2\alpha}$ would be luteolytic in man and could therefore be used as a post-coital contraceptive have not been realised. Nevertheless, prostaglandins can be used to induce termination during the early weeks of pregnancy. However, under these circumstances, abortion is often incomplete and may be accompanied by unpleasant side effects.

The E-series prostaglandins have a number of actions which are of potential therapeutic value. For example their vasodilatory action could be used to treat hypertension, their bronchodilatory action to treat asthma and their gastric antisecretory action to treat ulcers. However, the natural compounds produce all of those effects, together with many others, nonselectively, and it would be necessary to produce much more selective compounds in order to obtain useful drugs. To date, attempts to produce selective synthetic PGE analogues have not met with outstanding success.

Prostacyclin, in addition to its potential value as an antithrombotic, shares the ability of E-series prostaglandins to cause vasodilatation and to inhibit gastric acid secretion. Since prostacyclin, unlike E-series prostaglandins, does not produce nausea, vomiting and diarrhoea, it is possible that synthetic prostacyclin analogues might be of value as antihypertensive and antiulcer agents. Interestingly, results in experimental animals suggest that it is possible to obtain prostacyclin analogues which inhibit gastric acid secretion and which do not inhibit platelet aggregation or cause vasodilatation[27].

The therapeutic value of drugs that inhibit prostaglandin synthesis, the aspirin-like drugs, is well known. However, these compounds are nonselective in that they block formation of all prostaglandins and it is possible that more selective compounds might be advantageous. One approach to this problem might be to look for compounds that selectively block the formation of each of the different endoperoxide metabolites. An example of this approach, the development of selective thromboxane synthetase inhibitors, has already been described and it is possible that other selective synthesis inhibitors might be useful drugs. Another approach, and one which has proved highly successful in other areas, is the development of selective antagonists. At the present time relatively few prostaglandin antagonists are known, and most of those are of relatively low potency and specificity[28]. Nevertheless, there is no reason to believe that superior compounds should not be obtainable. Furthermore, since there are probably several different types of prostaglandin receptor, it should be possible to obtain several different classes of selective antagonist and this is an area which would probably repay closer study.

Further reading

There are a number of areas of prostaglandin research which have not been included in this chapter and the reader is referred to the many excellent reviews on these subjects. These include: prostaglandins and cancer[29]; prostaglandins in immunology and allergy[30,31]; prostaglandins and the regulation of adrenergic transmission[32]; and prostaglandins and the central nervous system[33].

References

1. N.H. ANDERSON and P.W. RAMWELL, *Archs. intern. Med.*, 1974, **30**, 133.
2. S.H. FERREIRA and J.R. VANE, *Nature, Lond.*, 1976, **216**, 869.
3. J. NAKANO, in *The Prostaglandins, Pharmacological and Therapeutic Advances*, Ed. M.F. Cuthbert, Heineman (London), 1973, p 23.
4. A. BENNETT, in *The Prostaglandins: Progress in Research*, Ed. S.M.M. Karim, John Wiley & Sons (New York), 1972, p 205.
5. S.M.M. KARIM and K. HILLIER, in *Prostaglandins and Reproduction*, Ed. S.M.M. Karim, Medical & Technical Publications (Lancaster), 1975, p 23.
6. A.P. SMITH and M.F. CUTHBERT, in *Advances in Prostaglandin and Thromboxane Research, vol. 1*, Eds. B. Samuelsson and R. Paoletti, Raven Press (New York) 1976, p 449.
7. J.R. VANE, *J. Allergy clin. Immunol.*, 1976, **58**, 691.
8. S.H. FERREIRA, *Nature, Lond.*, 1972, **240**, 200.
9. W. FELDBERG, in *Prostaglandin Synthetase Inhibitors*, Eds. H.J. Robinson and J.R. Vane, Raven Press (New York), 1974, p 197.
10. E.W. HORTON and N.L. POYSER, *Physiol. Rev.*, 1976, **56**, 595.
11. M. HAMBERG, J. SVENSSON, T. WAKABAYASHI and B. SAMUELSSON, *Proc. natn. Acad. Sci. U.S.A.*, 1974, **71**, 345.
12. D.H. NUGTEREN and E. HAZELHOFF, *Biochim. biophys. Acta*, 1973, **326**, 448.
13. S. MONCADA and J.R. VANE, *Pharmac. Rev.*, 1979, **30**, 293.
14. G.J. DUSTING, S. MONCADA and J.R. VANE, *Prostaglandins*, 1977, **13**, 3.
15. M. HAMBURG, P. HEDQVIST, K. STRANDBERG, J. SVENSSON and B. SAMUELSSON, *Life Sci.*, 1975, **16**, 451.
16. P. NEEDLEMAN, M. MINKES and A. RAZ, *Science, N.Y.*, 1976, **183**, 163.
17. D.F. REINGOLD and P. NEEDLEMAN, *TIPS*, 1980, **1**, 359.
18. R.L. JONES, in *Advances in Prostaglandin and Thromboxane Research, vol. 1*, Eds. B. Samuelsson and R. Paoletti, Raven Press (New York) 1976, p 221.
19. B.J.R. WHITTLE, S. MONCADA and J.R. VANE, *Prostaglandins*, 1978, **16**, 373.
20. P.J. PIPER and J.R. VANE, *Nature, Lond.*, 1969, **223**, 23.
21. M. HAMBERG, J. SVENSSON and B. SAMUELSSON, *Proc. natn. Acad. Sci. U.S.A.*, 1975, **72**, 2994.
22. J. SVENSSON, K. STRANDBERG, M. HAMBERG and B. SAMUELSSON, *Prostaglandins*, 1977, **14**, 425.
23. S. MONCADA, R. KORBUT, S. BUNTING and J.R. VANE, *Nature, Lond.*, 1978, **273**, 767.
24. R. KORBUT and S. MONCADA, *Thromb. Res.*, 1978, **13**, 489.
25. J.H. TURNEY, L.C. WILLIAMS, M.R. FEWELL, V. PARSONS and M.V. WESTON, *Lancet*, 1980, **ii**, 219.
26. J. DYERBERG, H.O. BANG, E. STOFFERSON, S. MONCADA and J.R. VANE, *Lancet*, 1978, **ii**, 117.
27. B.J.R. WHITTLE and N.K. BOUGHTON-SMITH, in *Prostacyclin*, Eds. J.R. Vane and S. Bergstrom, Raven Press (New York), 1979, p 159.
28. A. BENNETT, *Prog. Drug Res.*, 1974, **8**, 83.
29. G.C. EASTY and D.M. EASTY, *Cancer Treat. Rev.*, 1976, **3**, 217.
30. J. MORLEY, J.L. BEATS, M.A. BRAY and W. PAUL, *J. R. Soc. Med.*, 1980, **73**, 443.
31. L.M. PELVS and H.R. STRAUSSER, *Life Sci.*, 1977, **20**, 903.
32. K.V. MALIK, *Fedn Proc.*, 1978, **37**, 203.
33. F. COCEANI, *Archs intern. Med.*, 1974, **133**, 119.

CHAPTER 4

Synthesis of prostaglandins from polycyclic molecules

Roger F. Newton
Chemical Research Department, Glaxo Group Research, Ware, Hertfordshire
and
Stanley M. Roberts
Chemical Research Department, Glaxo Group Research, Greenford, Middlesex

Introduction

There are over fifty synthetic routes to prostaglandins that involve the use of polycyclic intermediates. We do not intend to comprehensively review this vast field of research since other texts are available which serve this purpose[1]. Instead we will concentrate on two synthetic routes, one developed in the laboratories at Harvard, and the other in the laboratories at Glaxo (Ware)[2]. These two routes illustrate that incorporating the five-membered ring of the prostaglandin into an inflexible molecule allows the introduction of the peripheral substituents in a stereocontrolled fashion.

The selected syntheses possess a number of advantages over many of the other pathways.

1. They lead to most of the classes of prostaglandin (A, C, D, E, F).
2. They provide prostaglandins of the natural configuration through a resolution step performed at an early stage in the synthetic sequence.

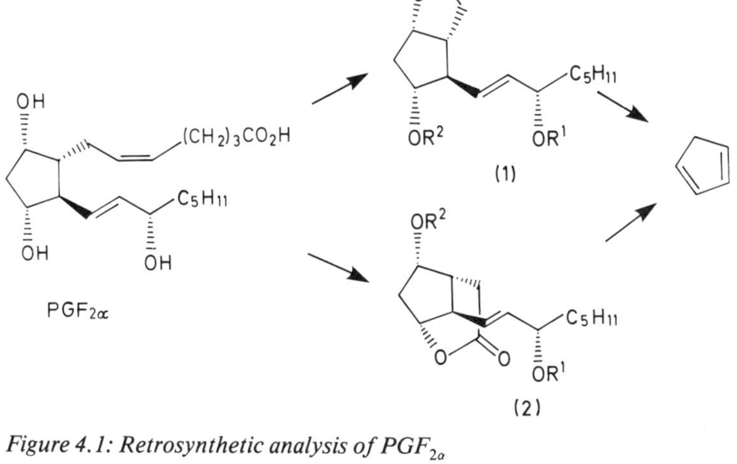

Figure 4.1: Retrosynthetic analysis of $PGF_{2\alpha}$

3. They involve high-yielding reactions using relatively simple reagents and conditions.
4. They can be readily adapted to furnish a range of analogues of the natural compounds.

Retrosynthetic analysis of the prostaglandin molecule (*see Figure 4.1*) suggests that the bicyclic molecules (1) and (2) would be desirable intermediates in prospective routes from a simple five-membered ring system such as cyclopentadiene.

Harvard synthesis

The Harvard route, engineered by Professor E.J. Corey, proceeds through the intermediacy of a lactone of type (1) as described in *Figure 4.2*. The various steps (i)–(xiii) are discussed in detail below.

2(i)

Tl

(a)

(b)

CH_2OCH_2Ph

(3)

Reagents :- (*a*) KOH, Tl_2SO_4; (*b*) $ClCH_2OCH_2Ph$, THF.

Alkylation of cyclopentadiene was accomplished by reacting the thallium salt with benzylchloromethyl ether at low temperature. These conditions minimized isomerization of the 5-substituted cyclopentadiene (3) to the 1- and 2-substituted compounds by 1,5-hydrogen shift(s).

2(ii)

CH_2OCH_2Ph

(3)

+

Cl COCl

CH_2OCH_2Ph

R

Cl

(4)

(a,b,c)

CH_2OCH_2Ph

O

(5)

Reagents :- (*a*) NaN_3, DME ; (*b*) heat ; (*c*) AcOH, H_2O.

Diels-Alder reaction of the diene (3) with 1-chloroacryloyl chloride gave the bicyclo[2.2.1]heptene (4; R = COCl) as a mixture of diastereoisomers having the 7-substituent *anti* to the carbon atom bearing the chloro-acid chloride functionality. Reaction of the acid chloride (4; R = COCl) with azide ion gave the corresponding acyl azide (4; R = CON_3) which underwent a Schmidt

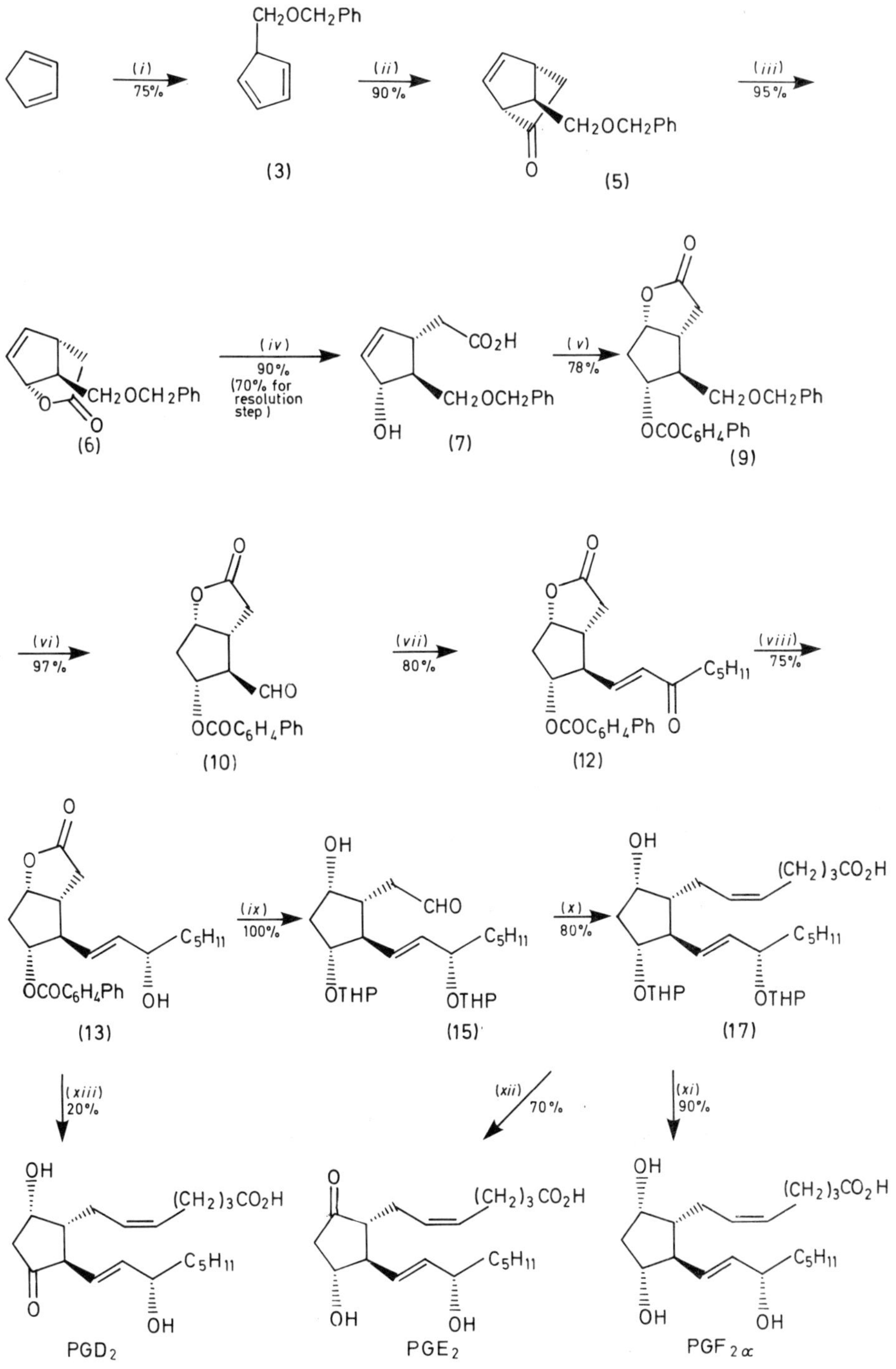

Figure 4.2: Synthesis of prostaglandins by Corey et al.

reaction on heating to give the isocyanate (4; R = NCO). Treatment with acetic acid at 60°C gave the required norbornanone (5).

2(iii)

(5) CH_2OCH_2Ph —(*a*)→ CH_2OCH_2Ph, OH, $OCOC_6H_4Cl$ —(*b*)→ (6) CH_2OCH_2Ph + $ClC_6H_4CO_2H$

Reagents:–(*a*) $ClC_6H_4CO_3H$, $NaHCO_3$, CH_2Cl_2.

Baeyer-Villiger oxidation of the ketone (5) proceeds through initial nucleophilic attack by the peracid at the carbonyl carbon atom to give a tetrahedral Criegee intermediate[3]. A 'rule of thumb' for the Baeyer-Villiger reaction suggests that the migratory alkyl group will be the one which is better able to support a positive charge. The allylic nature of C-1 leads to the lactone (6) being formed exclusively. The double bond is not epoxidized under the reaction conditions, being protected by the substituent at C-7.

2(vi)

(6) CH_2OCH_2Ph —(*a,b*)→ (7) CO_2H, CH_2OCH_2Ph, OH

Reagents:- (*a*) NaOH, H_2O; (*b*) CO_2.

The racemic lactone (6) furnished the hydroxyacid (7) on treatment with hydroxide ion: the hydroxyacid was resolved in a classic manner using (+)-amphetamine or L-arginine as the optically active base. The enantiomer of (7) was discarded.

2(v)

(7) CO_2H, CH_2OCH_2Ph, OH —(*a*)→ CH_2OCH_2Ph, OH →

(8) CH_2OCH_2Ph, OH —(*b*)→ CH_2OCH_2Ph, $OCOC_6H_4Ph$ —(*c*)→ (9) CH_2OCH_2Ph, $OCOC_6H_4Ph$

Reagents:- (*a*) KI, I_2, H_2O; (*b*) *p*-PhC_6H_4COCl, pyridine; (*c*) Bu_3SnH, C_6H_6.

Treatment of the acid (7) with iodine afforded the intermediate iodonium ion which suffered intramolecular nucleophilic attack to give, after deprotonation, the lactone (8). The hydroxyl group was protected as the *p*-phenylbenzoate ester: the advantage of using this moiety as the protecting group will become apparent in Section 2(viii). Hydrodeiodination with tri-n-butyltin hydride gave the lactone (9).

2(vi)

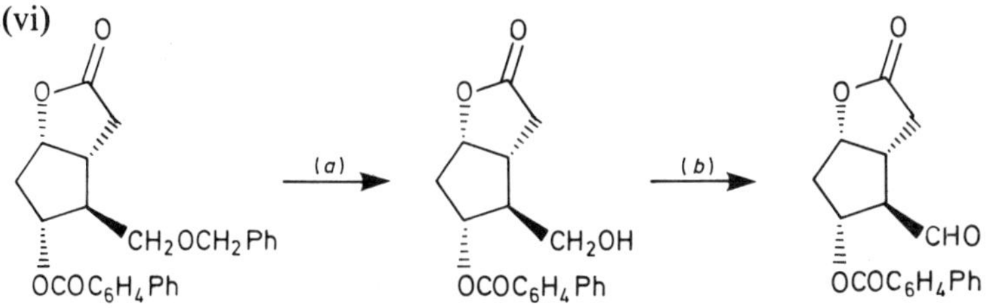

CH_2OCH_2Ph / $OCOC_6H_4Ph$ (9) —(a)→ CH_2OH / $OCOC_6H_4Ph$ —(b)→ CHO / $OCOC_6H_4Ph$ (10)

Reagents :- (*a*) H_2,Pd-C, EtOAc, EtOH, HCℓ; (*b*) CrO_3, pyridine, $CH_2Cℓ_2$

Debenzylation of the ether group in (9) was achieved in standard fashion by hydrogenolysis using a palladium catalyst. The primary alcohol was oxidized to the corresponding aldehyde (10) with Collins reagent (chromium trioxide in pyridine) or a chlorine/methyl phenyl sulphide complex.

2(vii)

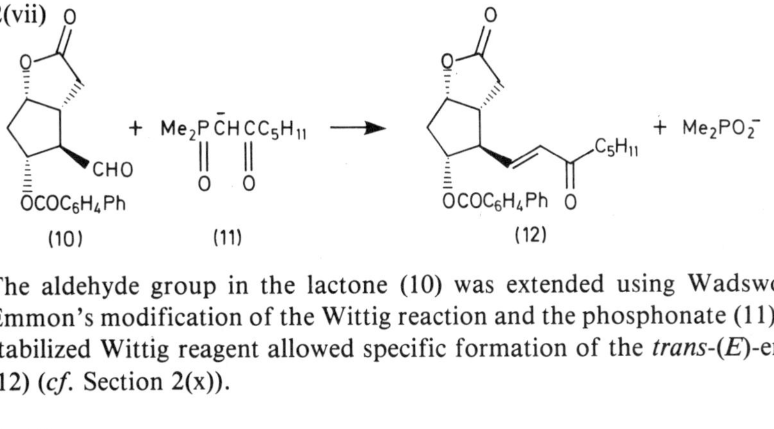

(10) CHO, $OCOC_6H_4Ph$ + $Me_2P(O)\bar{C}HC(O)C_5H_{11}$ (11) → (12) C_5H_{11}, $OCOC_6H_4Ph$ + $Me_2PO_2^-$

The aldehyde group in the lactone (10) was extended using Wadsworth-Emmon's modification of the Wittig reaction and the phosphonate (11): the stabilized Wittig reagent allowed specific formation of the *trans*-(*E*)-enone (12) (*cf.* Section 2(x)).

2(viii)

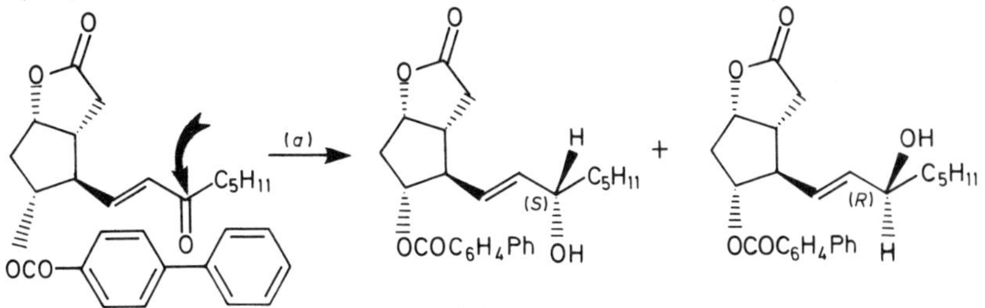

(12) C_5H_{11}, OCO– —(a)→ (13) H, C_5H_{11}, (S), $OCOC_6H_4Ph$, OH + OH, C_5H_{11}, (R), $OCOC_6H_4Ph$, H

Reagents :- (*a*) $LiB(Bu^s)_3H$.

The choice of the biphenyl ester group for hydroxyl group protection was due to its ability to hold the enone side chain of (12) in the *s-cis* conformation, as shown above, through hydrophobic and van der Waals interactions. The bulky borohydride reducing agent $LiBu^{S}_{3}BH$ preferentially attacked the carbonyl group from the less hindered face to give mainly the product with the required 15(*S*) configuration (13) [ratio 15(*S*):15(*R*) = 7:2 (prostaglandin numbering)]. Hence the 11-substituent of the prostaglandin intermediate is used to induce asymmetry at C-15. The lactone (13) was purified by chromatography.

2(ix)

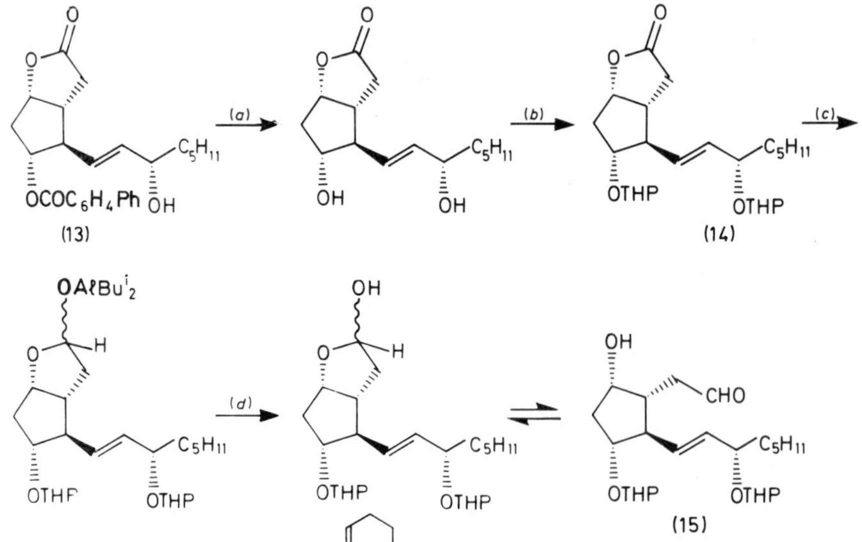

(13) → (a) → (b) → (14) → (c) → (d) ⇌ (15)

Reagents:- (*a*) K_2CO_3, MeOH; (*b*) dihydropyran, H^+, CH_2Cl_2; (*c*) $Bu^{i}_{2}AlH$; (*d*) H_2O.

The *p*-phenylbenzoate protecting group was removed from (13) using potassium carbonate in methanol and the base-stable, acid labile tetrahydropyranyl (THP) protecting group was appended using dihydropyran and an acid catalyst. Controlled reduction of the lactone was accomplished using di-isobutyl-aluminium hydride in a non-polar solvent. The first-formed aluminium salt was decomposed by water to give the lactol in equilibrium with a small amount of the hydroxyaldehyde (15).

2(x)

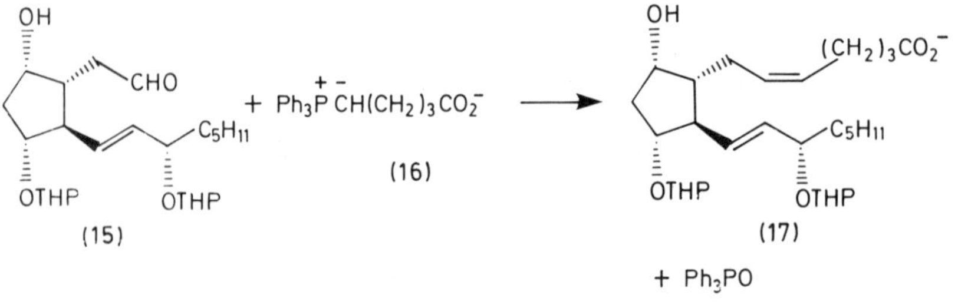

(15) + $Ph_3\overset{+}{P}\overset{-}{C}H(CH_2)_3CO_2^-$ (16) → (17) + Ph_3PO

The preferred kinetic product from the reaction of the aldehyde (15) with the phosphorane (16) is the *erythro* betaine (*see Figure 4.3*): isomerization to the thermodynamically favoured *threo* isomer (by proton abstraction from the active methine position and reprotonation *or* by breakdown of the *erythro*

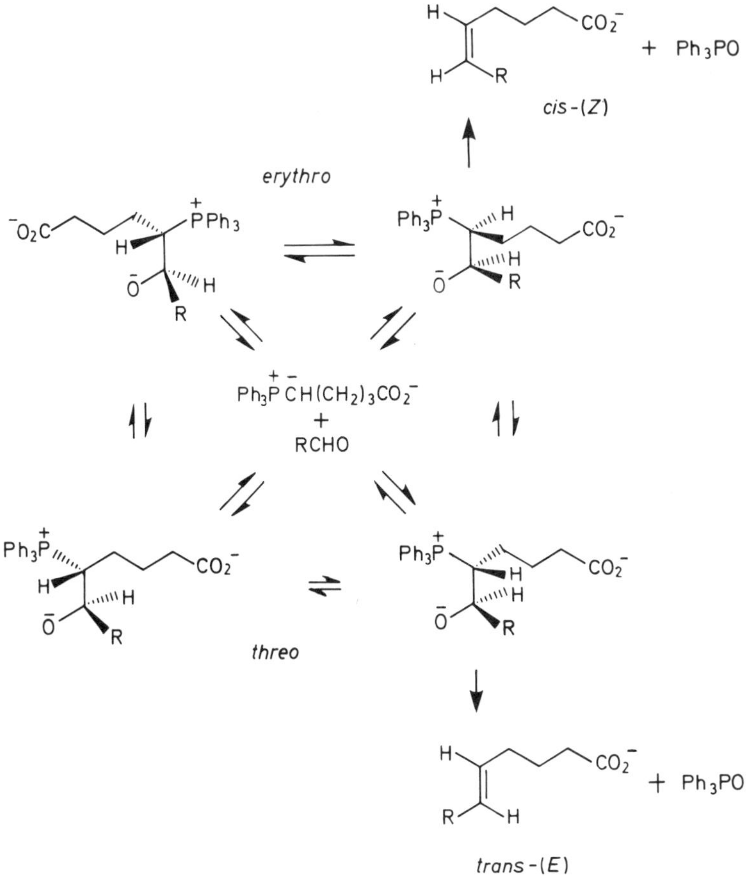

Figure 4.3: Stereochemistry of the Wittig reaction

adduct to the aldehyde and the phosphorane and recombination) can occur slowly. However, the *erythro-adduct is rendered unstable by conducting the reactions under 'salt-free'* conditions and rapidly loses triphenylphosphine oxide to give the *cis*-(*Z*)-alkene (17)[4].

2(xi)

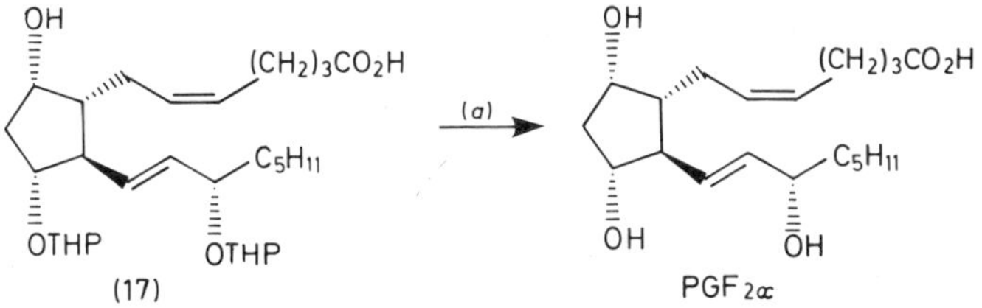

Reagents:- (*a*) AcOH, H_2O, 40 °C.

Acid catalyzed hydrolysis of the tetrahydropyranyl protecting groups from (17) gave crystalline prostaglandin $F_{2\alpha}$.

2(xii)

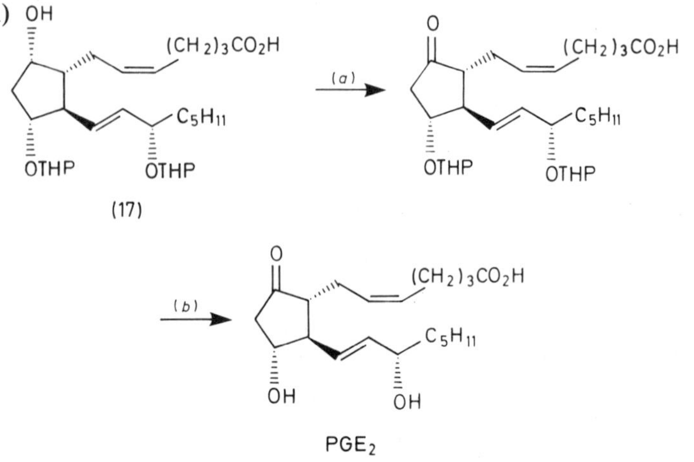

Reagents:- (*a*) Jones reagent; (*b*) AcOH, H_2O.

The 11,15-diprotected prostaglandin $F_{2\alpha}$ (17) was oxidized by Jones reagent under carefully controlled conditions to give the corresponding diprotected prostaglandin E_2. Acid catalyzed hydrolysis of the protecting groups gave prostaglandin E_2.

2(xiii)

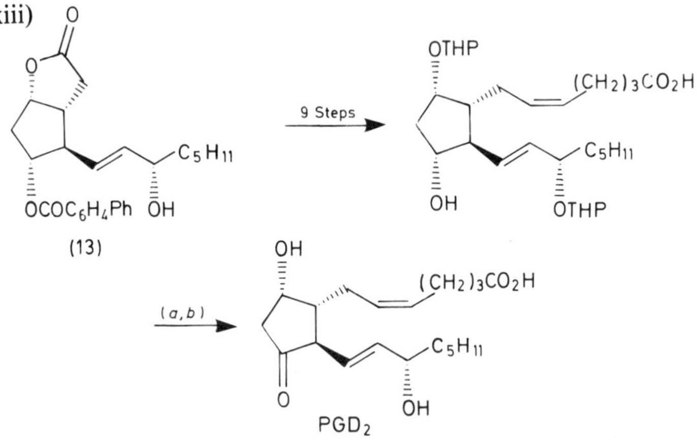

Reagents:- (*a*) Jones reagent; (*b*) AcOH, H_2O.

Access to the prostaglandin D series from the Harvard route is difficult and required a large number of interchanges of the protecting groups in order to form the desired 9,15-diprotected prostaglandin $F_{2\alpha}$ from the lactone (13); oxidation and deprotection gave prostaglandin D_2.

The Corey approach to prostaglandins of the A and C series is described in *Figure 4.4.* The starting material (18) was obtained by a Diels-Alder reaction

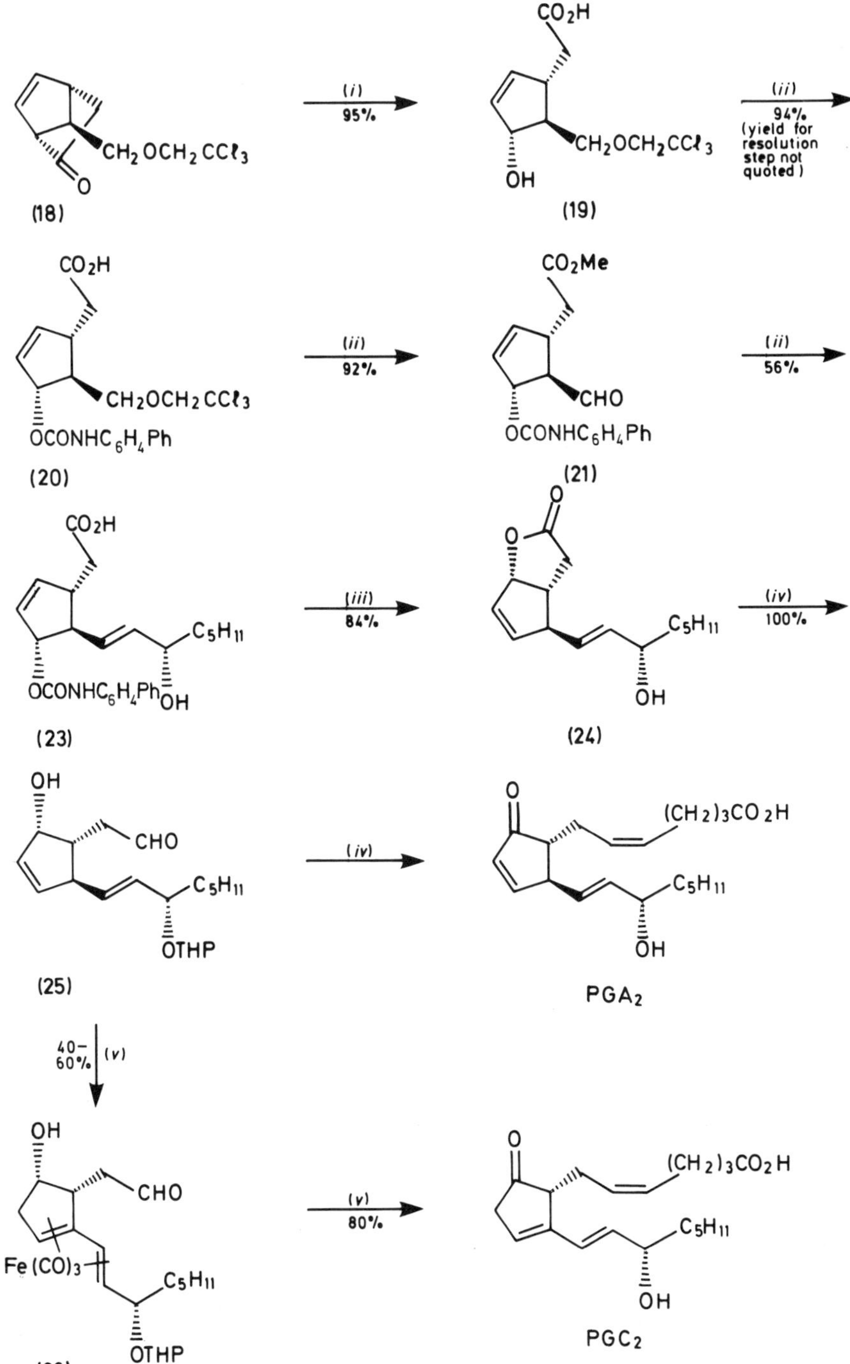

Figure 4.4: Corey synthesis of PGA_2 and PGC_2

on 5-trichloroethoxymethyl cyclopentadiene: the major difference in this strategy to that described in *Figure 4.2* is that the lower side-chain is developed prior to formation of the γ-lactone ring. Some key features in this sequence are described in *Sections 4(i)-4(v).*

4(i)

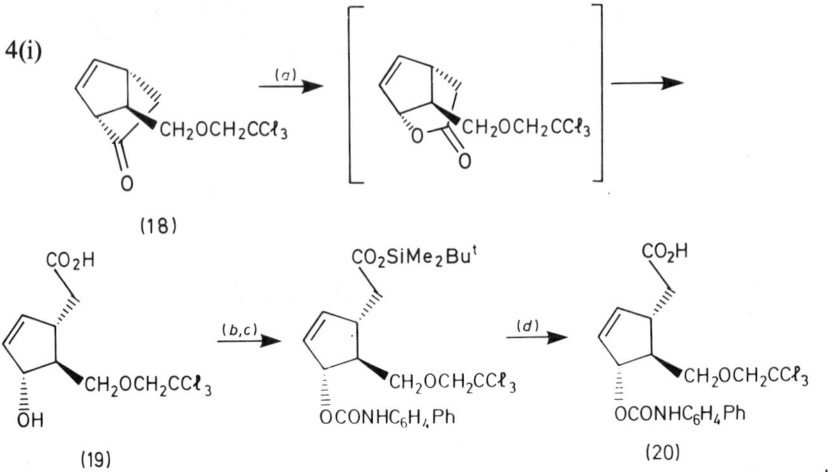

(18) (19) (20)

Reagents:- (*a*) H_2O_2, NaOH; (*b*) Bu^tMe_2SiCl; (*c*) *p*-PhC_6H_4NCO, Et_3N, THF; (*d*) H^+.

The ketone (18) was oxidized under basic conditions to give directly the required hydroxyacid (19), from which the carbamate (20) was formed in three steps. The latter compound was resolved using (+)-amphetamine.

4(ii)

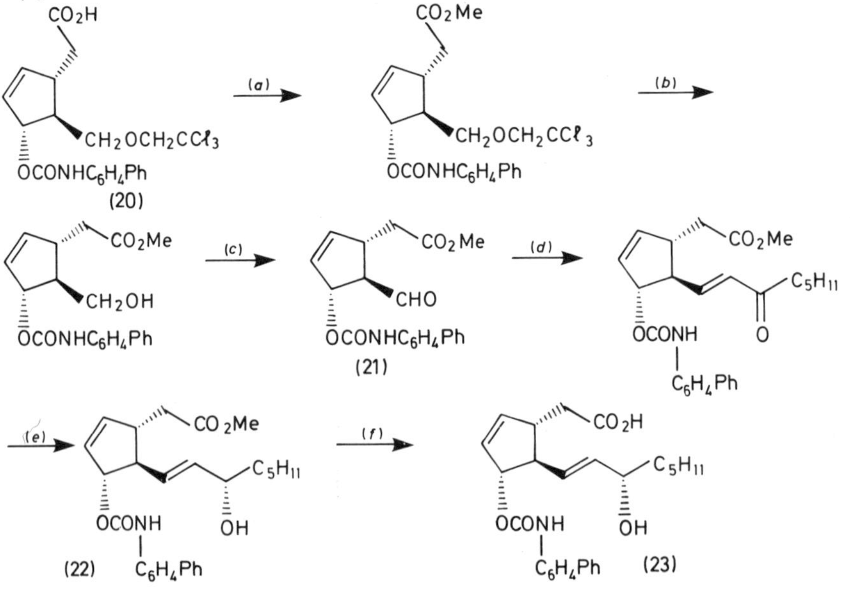

(20) (21) (22) (23)

Reagents:- (*a*) CH_2N_2; (*b*) Zn/Cu, MeOH, $ZnCl_2$; (*c*) Collins reagent; (*d*) sodium dimethyl 2-oxoheptylphosphonate; (*e*) $NaBHR_3$; (*f*) NaOH, THF, H_2O.

The carbamate (20) was esterified with diazomethane and the trichloroethyl moiety was removed using a zinc-copper couple. Collins oxidation of the primary hydroxyl function gave the corresponding aldehyde (21) which was subjected to a Wadsworth-Emmons-Wittig reaction involving sodio dimethyl 2-oxoheptylphosphonate. Trialkylborohydride reduction of the enone gave the required alkenol (22) contaminated with *ca.* 10 per cent of the 15-epimer. The ester group was hydrolyzed with base to give the hydroxyacid (23).

4(iii)

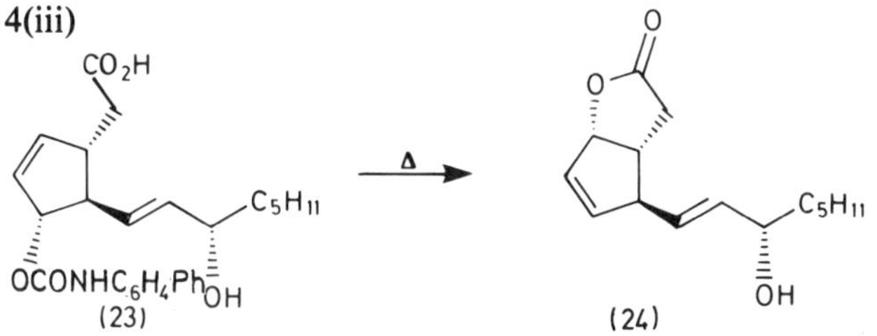

(23) → (24)

Heating a solution of acid (23) in aqueous dimethoxyethane buffered to pH 7 produced the lactone (24) in high yield.

4(iv)

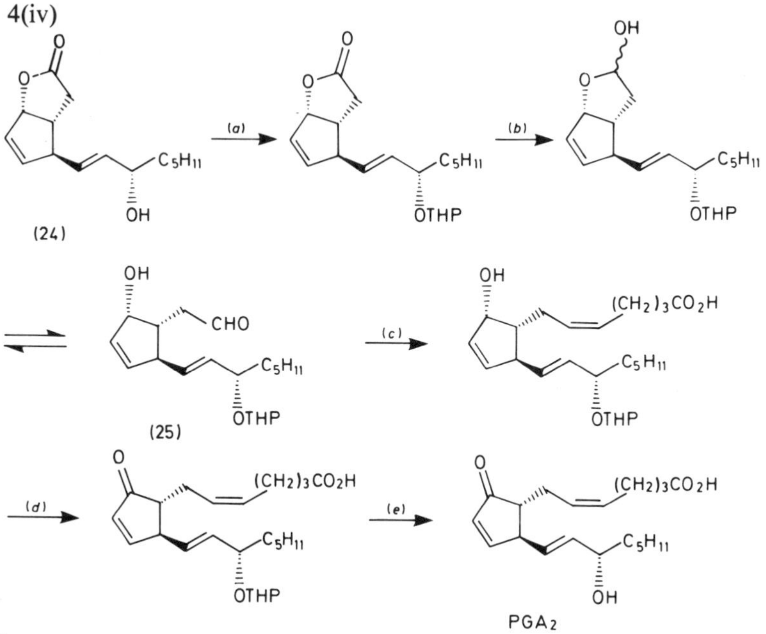

(24) → (25) → PGA_2

Reagents:- (*a*) DHP, *p*-TsOH; (*b*) Dibal, toluene; (*c*) 5-triphenylphosphoniopentanoic acid, sodium methylsulphinylmethylide, DMSO, (*d*) Collins oxidation; (*e*) AcOH, H_2O.

The synthesis of prostaglandin A_2 from (24) was completed in standard fashion. Thus the hydroxylactone (24) was converted into the corresponding tetrahydropyranyl ether, reduced to a mixture of the lactol and the hydroxyaldehyde (25), subjected to a 'salt-free' Wittig reaction, oxidized with Collins reagent, and deprotected to give (+)-prostaglandin A_2.

4(v)

(25) (26) PGC$_2$

Reagents:- (*a*) $Fe_3(CO)_{12}$, DME; (*b*) 5-triphenylphosphoniopentanoic acid, sodium methylsulphinylmethylide, DMSO; (*c*) Collins reagent; (*d*) AcOH, H_2O

Treatment of the diene (25) with triiron dodecacarbonyl gave the stable iron-carbonyl complex (26). The upper side chain was developed using a Wittig reaction in the usual way. The iron was then removed by reaction with excess Collins reagent, which also served to oxidize the ring hydroxyl group. The 15-protected prostaglandin C_2 was treated carefully with aqueous acetic acid to remove the tetrahydropyranyl protecting group without causing isomerization to prostaglandin B_2.

Glaxo synthesis

The major features of the Glaxo synthesis are shown in *Figure 4.5*. It can be seen that lactones of types (1) and (2) (*see Figure 4.1*) are involved and that

(*i*) 70% (27) (*ii*) 77% (28) (32) (29) (*iii*) 42% (*v*) 70% (35% for resolution step) (*iv*) 94% (30) (33) (31)

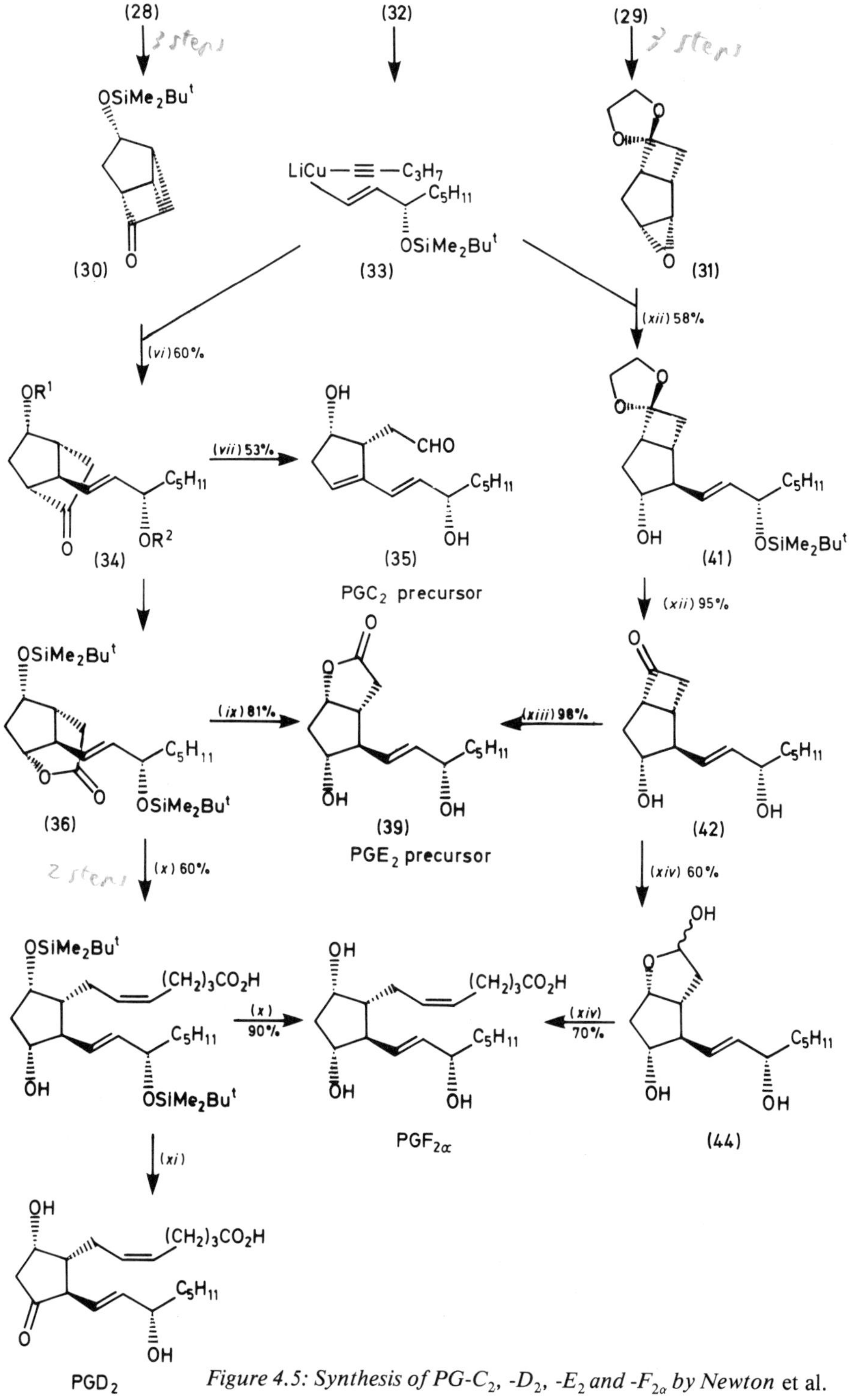

(28)

$OSiMe_2Bu^t$

(30)

(32)

$LiCu—≡—C_3H_7$

C_5H_{11}

$OSiMe_2Bu^t$

(33)

(29)

(31)

(vi) 60%

OR^1

C_5H_{11}

OR^2

(34)

(vii) 53%

OH

CHO

C_5H_{11}

OH

(35)

PGC_2 precursor

(xii) 58%

C_5H_{11}

OH

$OSiMe_2Bu^t$

(41)

(xii) 95%

$OSiMe_2Bu^t$

C_5H_{11}

$OSiMe_2Bu^t$

(36)

(ix) 81%

C_5H_{11}

OH

OH

(39)

PGE_2 precursor

(xiii) 98%

C_5H_{11}

OH

OH

(42)

(x) 60%

(xiv) 60%

$OSiMe_2Bu^t$

$(CH_2)_3CO_2H$

C_5H_{11}

OH

$OSiMe_2Bu^t$

(x) 90%

OH

$(CH_2)_3CO_2H$

C_5H_{11}

OH

OH

$PGF_{2\alpha}$

(xiv) 70%

OH

C_5H_{11}

OH

OH

(44)

(xi)

OH

$(CH_2)_3CO_2H$

C_5H_{11}

OH

PGD_2

Figure 4.5: Synthesis of PG-C_2, -D_2, -E_2 and -$F_{2\alpha}$ by Newton et al.

prostaglandin D_2 as well as prostaglandin E_2, prostaglandin C_2 and $F_{2\alpha}$ are readily available from one or both of the enantiocomplementary routes. Some details of this work are given in *Sections 5(i)–5(xiv).*

5(i)

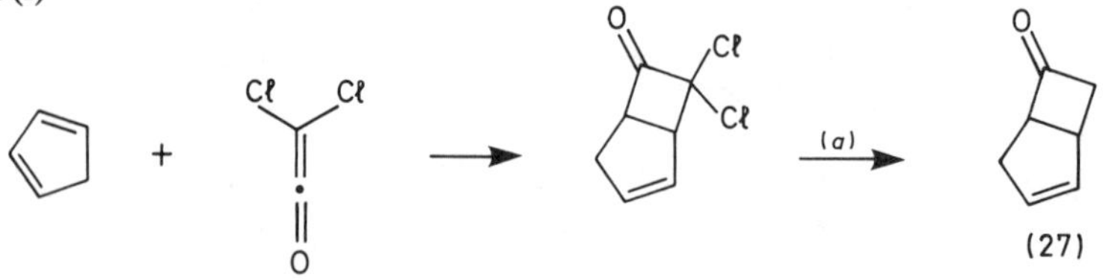

(27)

Reagents :- (*a*) Zn, AcOH.

Cyclopentadiene reacted readily with dichloroketen in a regiospecific manner. Dichloroketen was used in the cycloaddition reaction because it is much more reactive than keten itself. Hydrodechlorination to give the bicycloheptenone (27) was achieved using zinc in acetic acid.

5(ii)

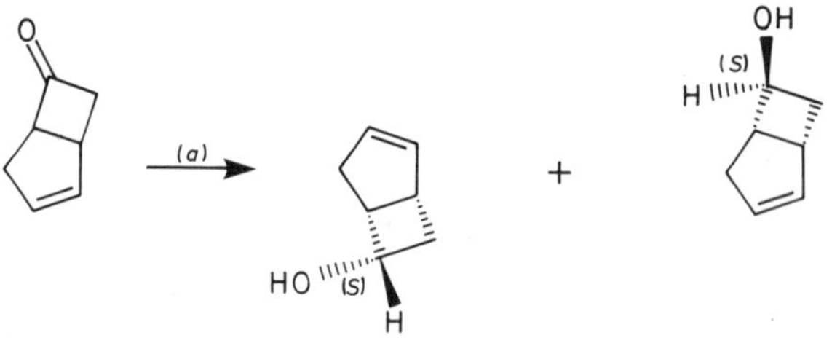

(27) (28) (29)

Reagents :- (*a*) yeast, glucose, H_2O, yeast nutrient.

The racemic ketone (27) was reduced by a dehydrogenase enzyme in actively fermenting yeast[5]. Steam distillation afforded the two alcohols (28) and (29) in high optical purity (greater than 85 per cent) and in good chemical yield and these were separated by distillation. Obviously the enzyme can only accept the enantiomeric ketones in the manner shown in *Figure 4.6* to give the (*S*)-configuration about the newly formed asymmetric centre in both cases.

5(iii)

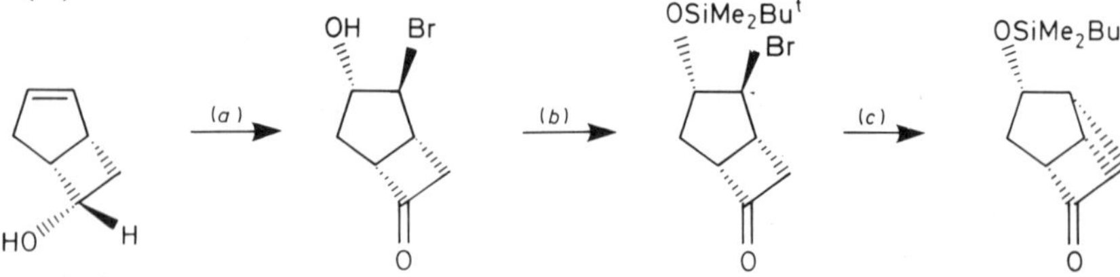

(28) (30)

Reagents: (*a*) *N*-Bromosuccinimide, H_2O, Me_2CO, AcOH; (*b*) $Bu^tMe_2SiC\ell$, imidazole, DMF; (*c*) $KOBu^t$, ether.

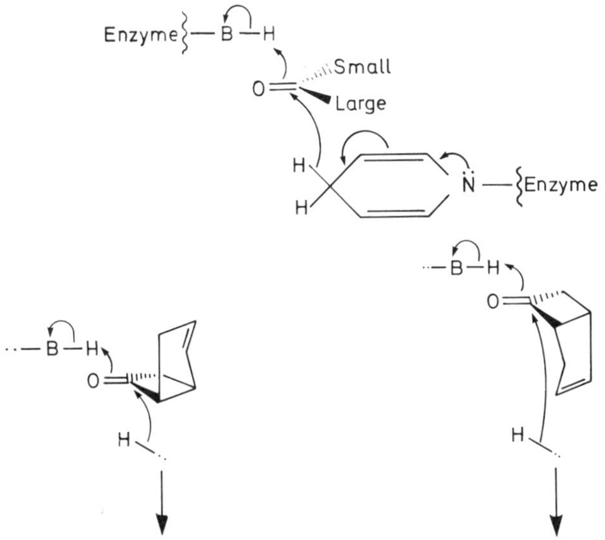

Figure 4.6: Reduction of bicyclo[3.2.0]hept-2-en-6-one using fermenting baker's yeast

Treatment of the alcohol (28) with *N*-bromosuccinimide or *N*-bromoacetamide in aqueous acetone caused oxidation of the secondary alcohol as well as functionalization of the double bond. Addition of HOBr across the alkene unit is remarkably selective due to the fixed, angular shape

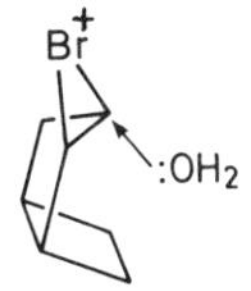

Figure 4.7: Preferred mode of bromohydroxylation of the bicyclo[3.2.0]hept-2-ene series

of the bicyclic molecule. Thus, bromonium ion formation took place exclusively on the exposed *exo*-face of the molecule and subsequent attack by water occurred at the relatively unhindered 3-position (*see Figure 4.7*). The bromohydrin was protected as the t-butyldimethylsilyl ether before base catalyzed dehydrobromination was effected by an intramolecular S_N2 reaction to give the tricyclic ketone (30).

5(iv)

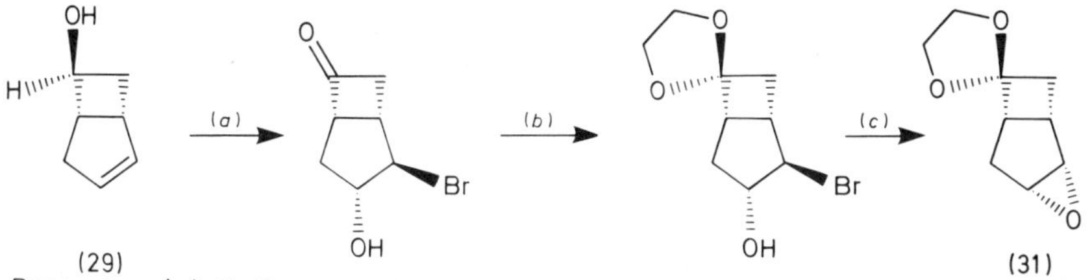

Reagents: (*a*) *N*-Bromosuccinimide, H_2O, Me_2CO, AcOH; (*b*) $(CH_2OH)_2$, H^+; (*c*) K_2CO_3, MeOH.

The bicycloheptenol (29) was converted into the corresponding bromohydroxyketone as discussed in *Section 5(iii)*. The carbonyl group was protected in standard fashion whereupon treatment with base furnished the epoxide (31).

5(v)

(32) → (33)

Reagents:- (*a*) phthalic acid, then (+)-phenethylamine, then crystallize, then H^+; (*b*) Bu^tMe_2SiCl, DMF, imidazole; (*c*) Bu^n_3SnH; (*d*) I_2; (*e*) Bu^nLi; (*f*) copper pentyne.

Racemic octyn-3-ol (32) was resolved in classical fashion through formation of the half phthalate ester and fractional crystallization of the salt formed with (+)-phenylethylamine. The hydroxyl group was protected as the t-butyldimethylsilyl ether before *syn*-addition of tri-n-butyltin hydride to the alkyne bond was carried out. Iodination, halogen-lithium exchange and reaction of the resultant alkenyllithium with copper pentyne gave the required cuprate reagent (33).

5(vi)

(30) —reagent (33), −78 °C→ (34, $R^1 = R^2 = SiMe_2Bu^t$)

Within the cuprate reagent (33) the copper alkene bond is much weaker than the copper alkyne bond: the alkene unit is preferentially transferred to the strained and highly reactive ketone (30) in a regiospecific homoconjugate addition reaction to give the bicyclo[2.2.1]heptanone (34, $R^1 = R^2 = SiMe_2Bu^t$).

5(vii)

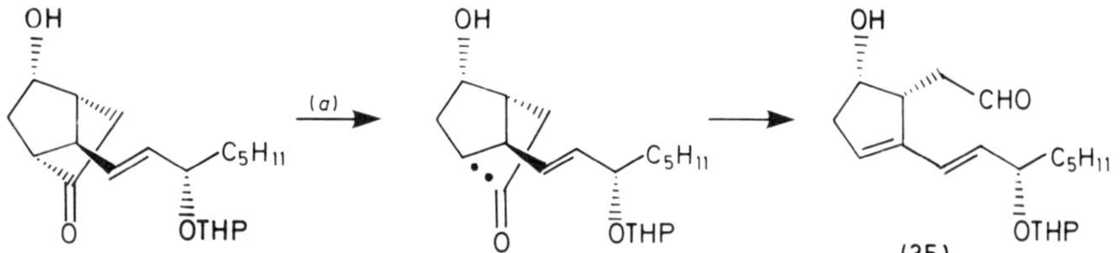

(34, $R^1 = H$; $R^2 = THP$) (35)

Reagents :- (*a*) $h\nu$, MeOH.

The bicyclic ketone (34, $R^1 = H$, $R^2 = THP$) was synthesized by a procedure analogous to that used for the preparation of the bis-silylated compound (34, $R^1 = R^2 = SiMe_2Bu^t$). Photolysis of the former ketone in methanol caused Norrish type I cleavage to furnish an acyl-alkyl diradical[6]. The acyl radical abstracted the adjacent hydrogen atom to give directly the prostaglandin C_2 precursor (35) [*see Section 4(v)*] in good yield.

5(viii)

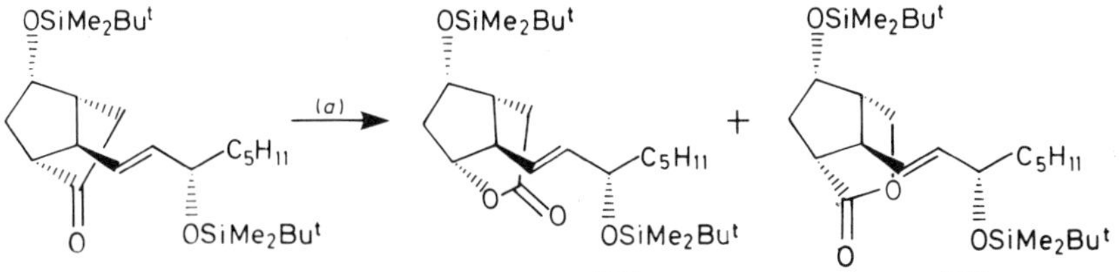

(34, $R^1 = R^2 = SiMe_2Bu^t$) (36) (37)

Reagents :- (*a*) $MeCO_3H$, $MeCO_2H$.

Baeyer-Villiger oxidation of the ketone (34; $R^1 = R^2 = SiMe_2Bu^t$) was nonspecific. Small amounts of the lactone (37) were produced together with the required product (36). However, the isomer (37) reacted readily with hydroxide ion while the lactone (36) was relatively stable, reflecting the different steric interactions within the two transition states (*see Figure 4.8*). The ring opened hydroxy acid and the prostaglandin precursor (36) were readily separated.

5(ix)

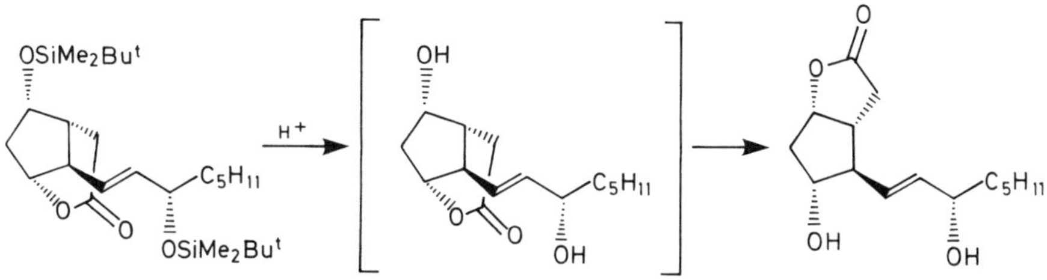

(36) $\xrightarrow{H^+}$ [(38)] $\rightarrow$ (39)

The t-butyldimethylsilyl protecting groups were removed from the lactone (36) under acidic conditions to give the unstable dihydroxy-δ-lactone (38) which rearranged spontaneously to the isomeric γ-lactone (39), a precursor of prostaglandin E_2 (*see Sections 2(ix), (x), (xii)).*

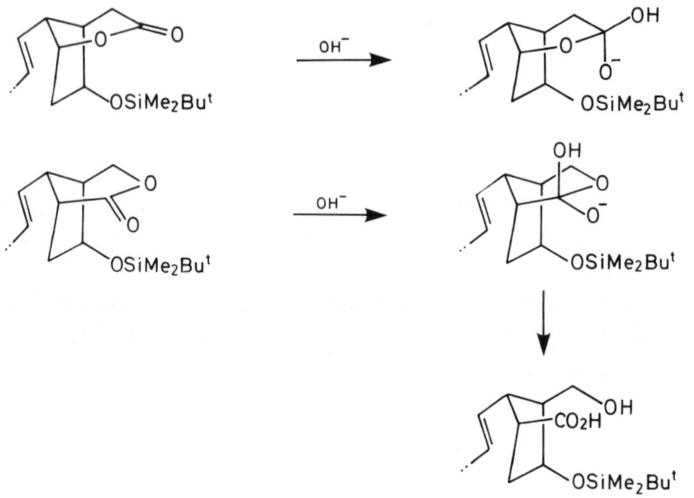

Figure 4.8: Selective hydrolysis of two δ-lactone isomers

5(x)

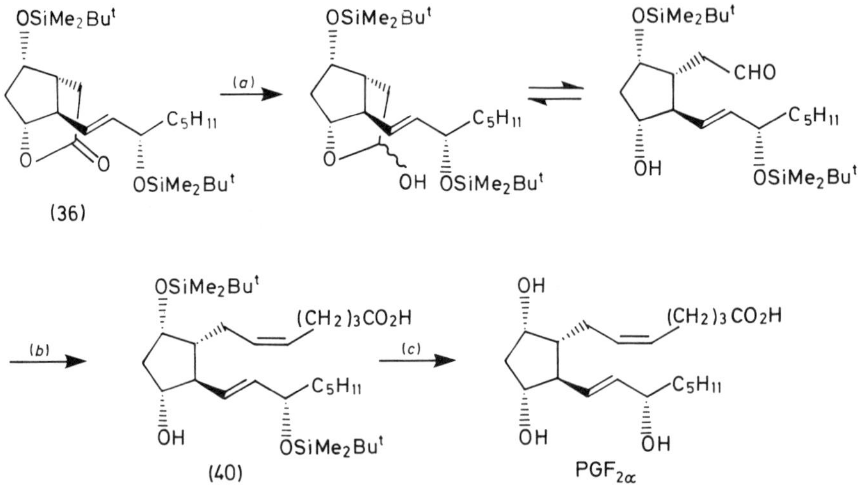

Reagents :- (*a*) Bu^i_2AlH; (*b*) 5-triphenylphosphoniopentanoic acid, sodium methylsulphinylmethylide, DMSO; (*c*) AcOH, H_2O.

The lactone (36) was reduced with di-isobutylaluminium hydride to give (after aqueous work up) the corresponding lactol/hydroxyaldehyde which was converted into the 9,15-diprotected prostaglandin $F_{2\alpha}$ (40) using the requisite Wittig reagent under 'salt-free' conditions. The silyl protecting groups on (40) were removed using aqueous acetic acid to give prostaglandin $F_{2\alpha}$.

5(xi)

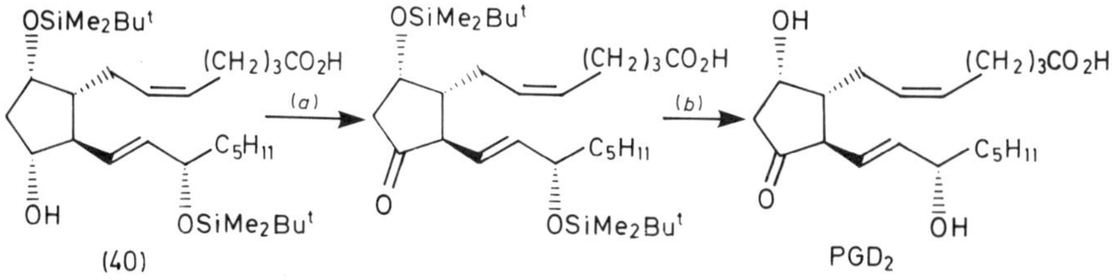

Reagents:- (*a*) Collins reagent ; (*b*) HF, H_2O, MeCN.

The free hydroxyl group in the prostanoid (40) was cleanly oxidized using pyridinium chlorochromate. Aqueous hydrofluoric acid in acetonitrile was the reagent of choice for the subsequent removal of the silyl protecting groups. The weak acidity of HF ($pK_a = 3.6$) combined with the high silicophilicity of the fluoride anion ensured rapid desilylation without concurrent dehydration of the β-ketol system of prostaglandin D_2.

5(xii)

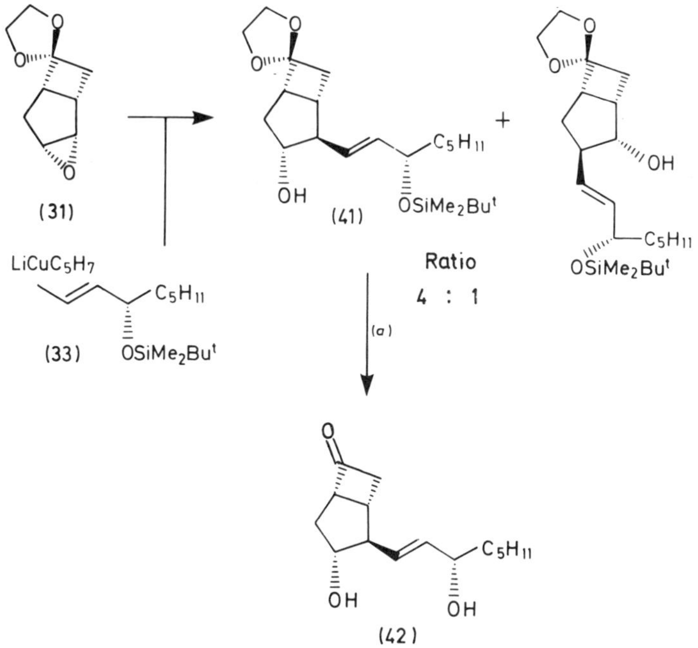

Reagents:- (*a*) H_2SO_4, H_2O.

The epoxide ring in the acetal (31) was opened by the cuprate reagent (33) in a very selective manner. The alkenylation obviously proceeds through the transition state which minimizes the highly unfavourable interaction between the developing oxyanion and the adjacent four-membered ring system (*see Figure 4.9*).

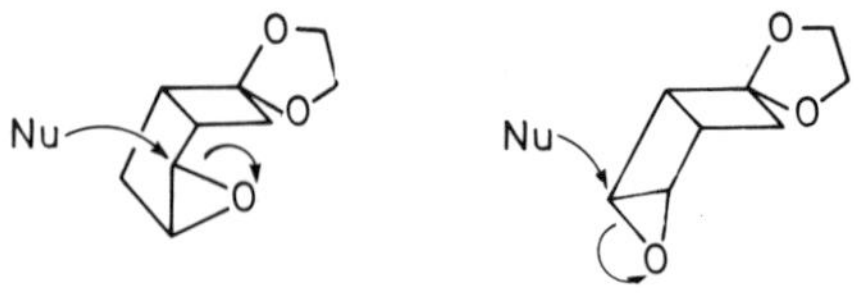

Nu
Nu
Favoured
Disfavoured

Figure 4.9: Selectivity in the ring-opening of a tricyclic intermediate

The prostaglandin precursor (41) was purified by column chromatography and deprotected using dilute sulphuric acid to give the dihydroxyketone (42).

5(xii)

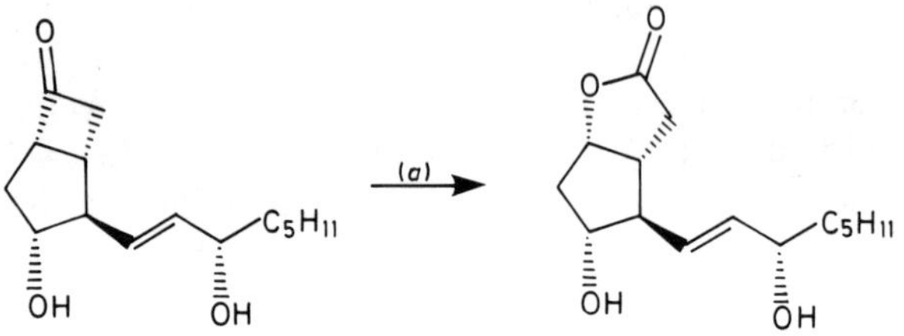

(42) —(a)→ (39)

Reagents:- (a) $NaHCO_3$, $ClC_6H_4CO_3H$, CH_2Cl_2

Baeyer-Villiger oxidation of the ketone (42) at low temperature gave the prostaglandin E_2 precursor (39).

5(xiv)

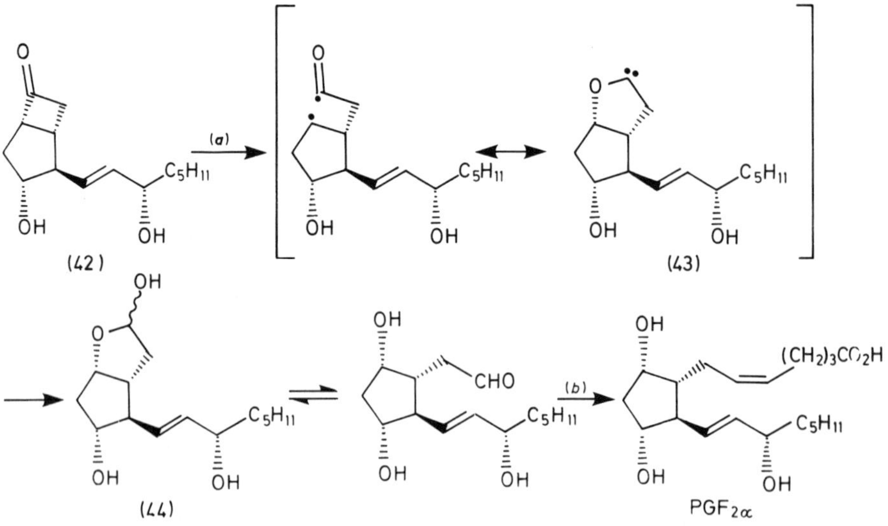

(42) —(a)→ [⟷ (43)] → (44) ⇌ —(b)→ $PGF_{2\alpha}$

Reagents:- (a) $h\nu$, H_2O, MeCN; (b) 5-triphenylphosphoniopentanoic acid, sodium methylsulphinylmethylide, DMSO.

Photolysis of the cyclobutanone derivative (42) caused Norrish Type I cleavage and formation of the oxacarbene (43) which was hydrated to give the γ-lactol (44)[7]. A Wittig reaction on (44) under the usual conditions gave prostaglandin $F_{2\alpha}$.

The Glaxo group have prepared prostaglandin A_2 from the bicycloheptenols (28) and (29) as described in *Figure 4.10.* Some key features of these routes are noted in *Sections 9(i)-9(viii).*

9(i)

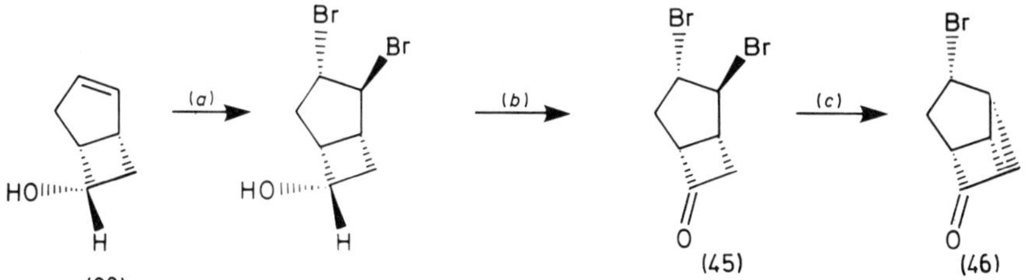

(28) → (a) → (b) → (45) → (c) → (46)

Reagents :- (*a*) Br_2, CCl_4, $NaHCO_3$; (*b*) Jones oxidation; (*c*) $KOBu^t$, ether.

Bromination of the optically active bicycloheptenol (28) followed by Jones oxidation gave the dibromobicycloheptanone (45) which was dehydrobrominated using potassium-tert-butoxide to give the crystalline ketone (46).

9(ii)

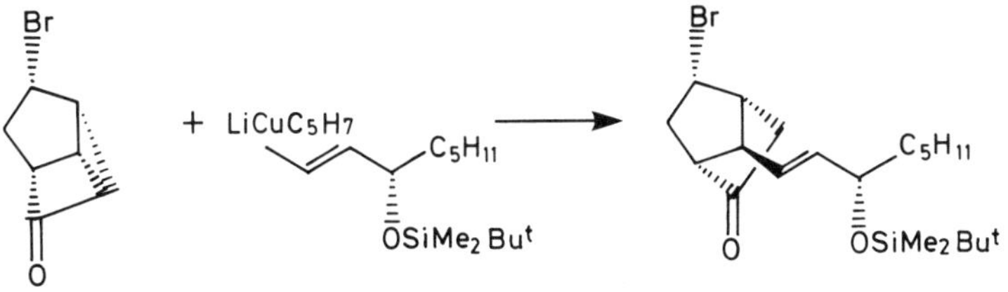

(46) + $LiCuC_5H_7$ (33) → (47)

The cuprate reagent (33) reacted with the bromoketone (46) to give the bicyclic ketone (47) as the only isolated product.

9(iii)

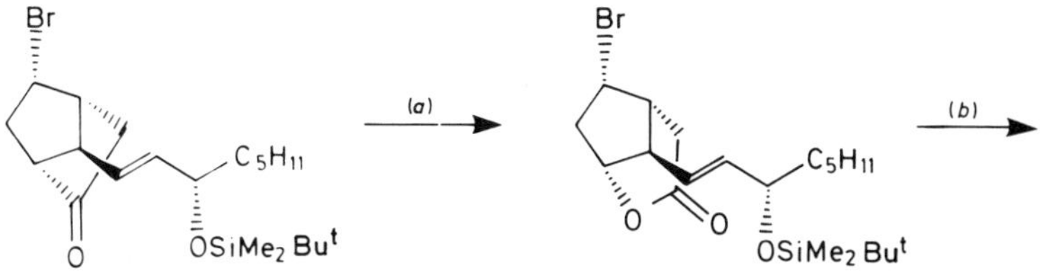

(47) → (a) → (48) → (b) →

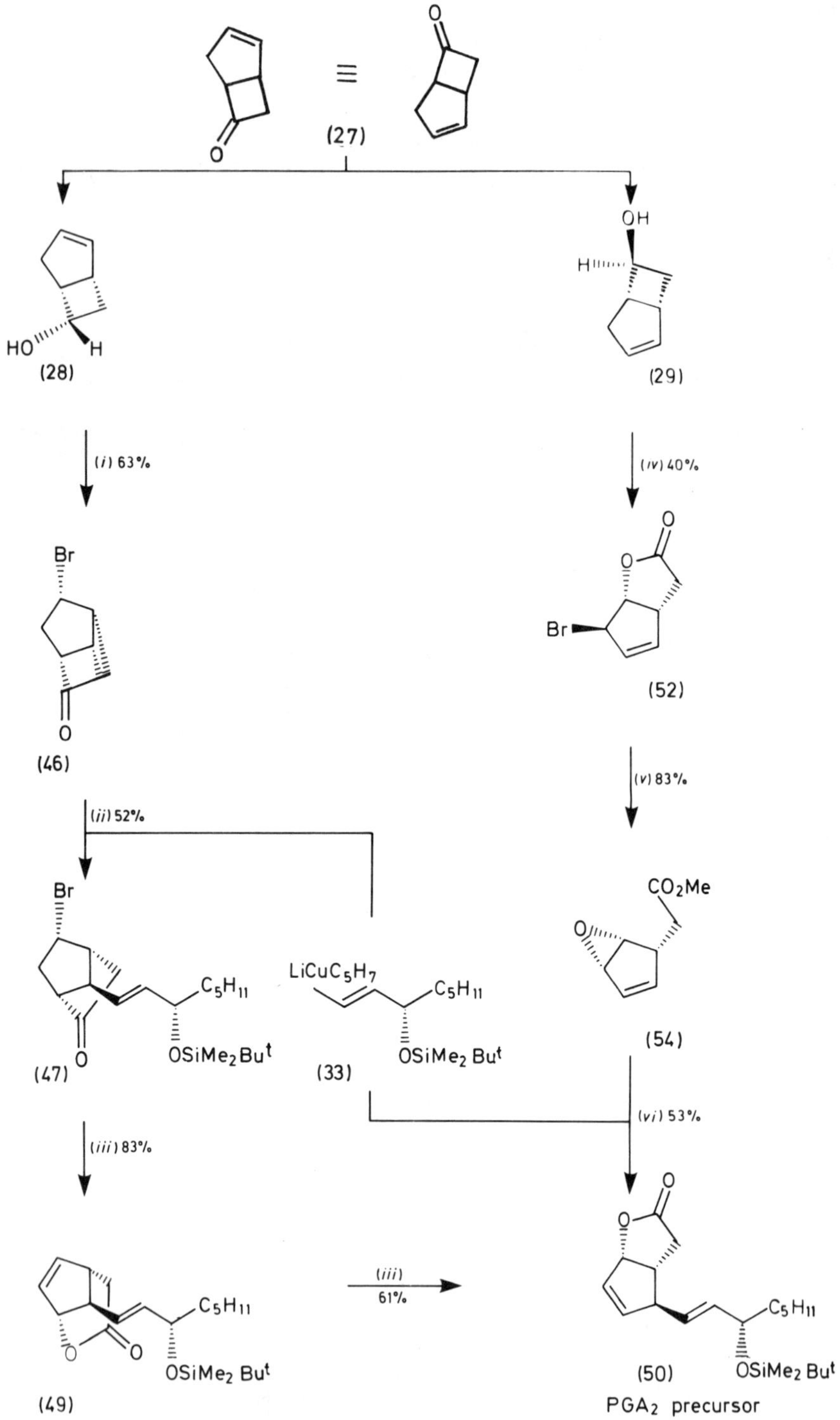

≡

(27)

OH

H

HO H

(28)

(29)

(i) 63%

(iv) 40%

Br

O

O

Br

(52)

O

(46)

(v) 83%

(ii) 52%

Br

CO_2Me

O

C_5H_{11}

$LiCuC_5H_7$

C_5H_{11}

O

$OSiMe_2Bu^t$

$OSiMe_2Bu^t$

(54)

(47)

(33)

(vi) 53%

(iii) 83%

O

O

(iii)

61%

C_5H_{11}

C_5H_{11}

O

O

$OSiMe_2Bu^t$

(50)

$OSiMe_2Bu^t$

(49)

PGA_2 precursor

Figure 4.10: Glaxo synthesis of PGA_2

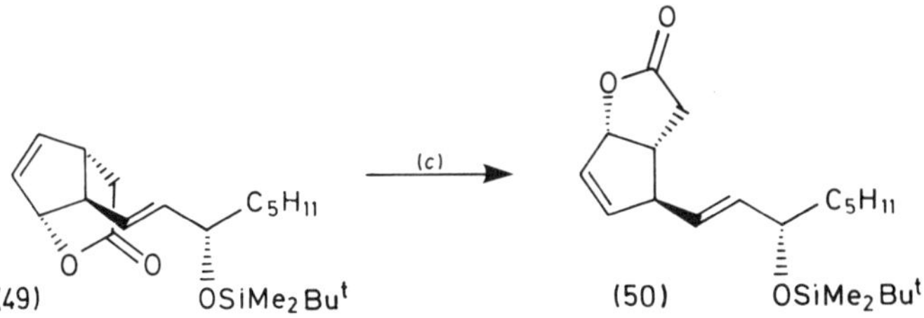

(49) (50)

Reagents:- (*a*) $ClC_6H_4CO_3H$, $NaHCO_3$, $MeCl_2$; (*b*) diazabicycloundecene, toluene; (*c*) DMF, heat.

Oxidation of the ketone (47) was accomplished in a highly regioselective fashion using *meta*-chloroperoxybenzoic acid to give the bromolactone (48). Dehydrobromination of (48) was accomplished using diazabicycloundecene (DBU) to give the unsaturated δ-lactone (49), which rearranged to the γ-lactone (50) on standing in hot dimethylformamide. Trace quantities of dimethylamine present in the latter solvent are responsible for this rearrangement as shown in *Figure 4.11*. The γ-lactone (50) was converted into prostaglandin A_2 as described above (*see Section 4(iv)*).

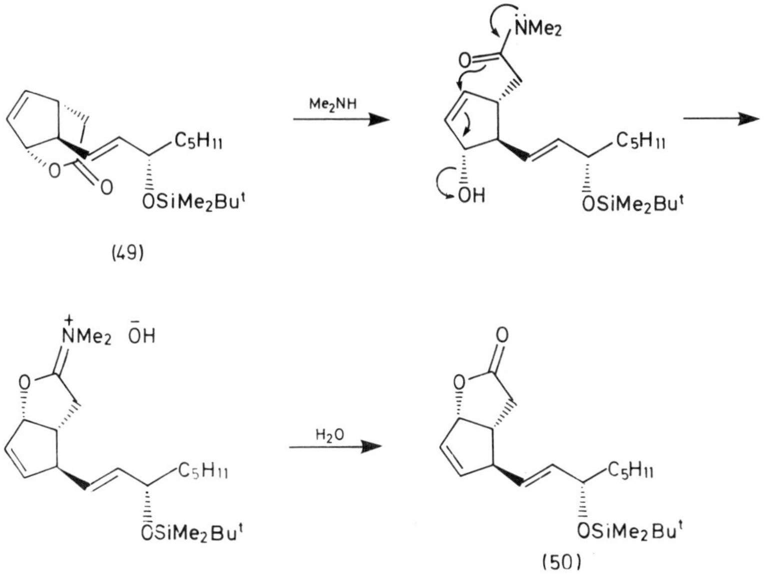

(49) (50)

Figure 4.11: Isomerization of a δ-lactone into a γ-lactone

The chiral bicycloheptenol (29) was oxidized to the unsaturated γ-lactone (51) by sequential Jones and Baeyer-Villiger oxidations. The required 8-bromolactone (52) was obtained by treating the lactone (51) with *N*-bromosuccinimide in carbon tetrachloride under floodlamp irradiation. The 6-bromolactone (53) was obtained as a minor impurity and was removed by chromatography.

9(iv)

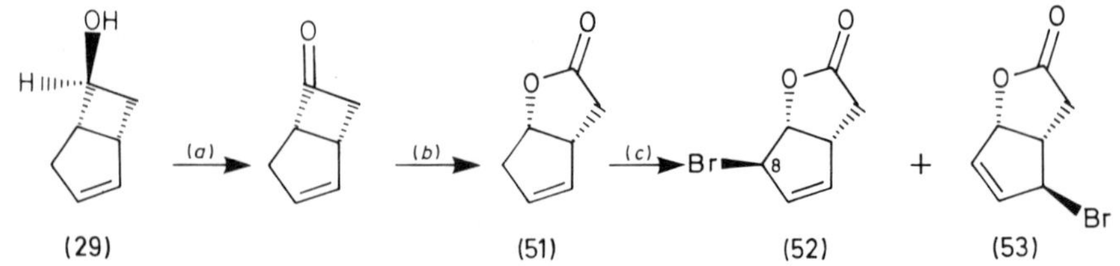

(29) (51) (52) (53)

Reagents:- (*a*) Jones oxidation; (*b*) $MeCO_3H$, $MeCO_2H$; (*c*) *N*-bromosuccinimide, CCl_4, *hν*

9(v)

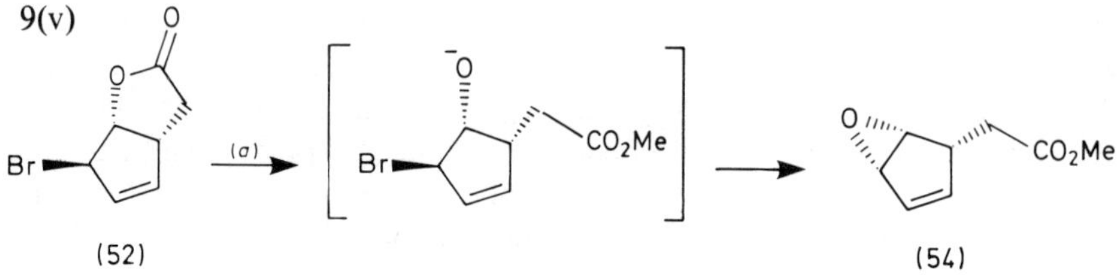

(52) (54)

Reagents:- (*a*) K_2CO_3, MeOH, Et_2O.

The bromolactone (52) furnished the epoxyester (54) on heating in ether and methanol containing potassium carbonate.

9(vi)

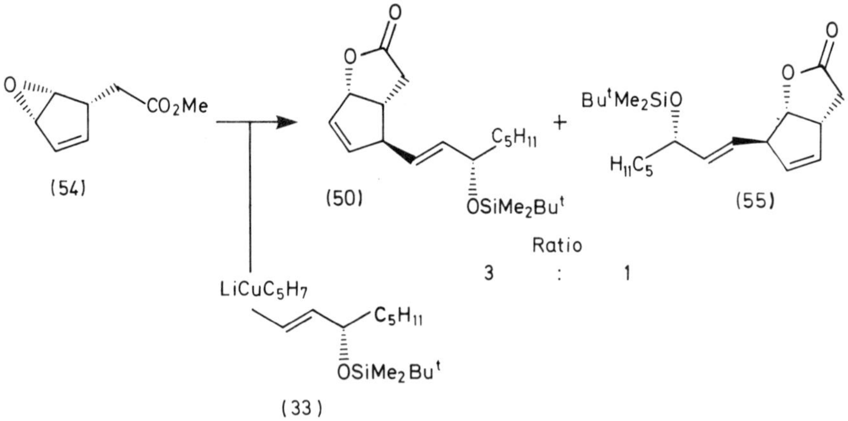

(54) (50) (55)

Ratio 3 : 1

(33)

The cuprate reagent (33) reacted with the epoxyester (54) in an $S_{N'}$ manner preferentially. The prostaglandin precursor (50) was contaminated with the product of an initial S_N2 displacement but this compound (55) was removed readily by chromatography. The $S_{N'}$ displacement with inversion of configuration that is observed in going from (54) to (50) is believed to proceed through initial formation of a copper (III) intermediate (*see Figure 4.12*)[8].

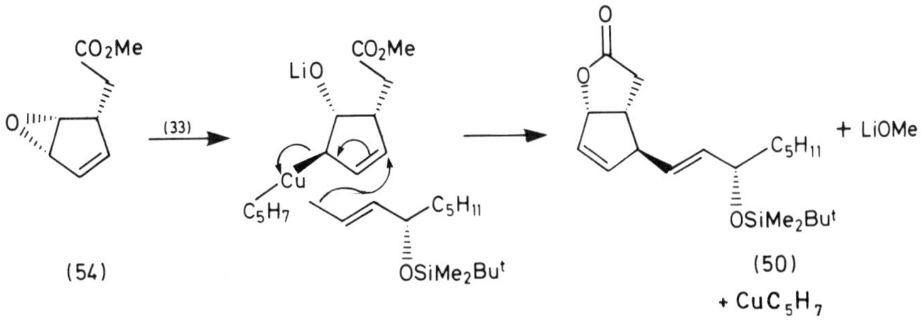

Figure 4.12. Reaction of an epoxy-ester with a cuprate agent.

References

1. J.S. BINDRA and R. BINDRA, *Prostaglandin synthesis,* Academic Press (New York), 1977; A. Mitra, *The Synthesis of Prostaglandin Derivatives,* John Wiley & Sons (New York), 1978; C. Szartay and L. Novak, *Synthesis of Prostaglandins*, Akademiai Kiado (Budapest), 1978.
2. R.F. NEWTON and S.M. ROBERTS, *Tetrahedron,* 1980, **36,** 2163.
3. R. CRIEGEE, *Annalen*, 1948, **560,** 127; J.B. Lee and B.C. Uff, *Q. Rev.,* 1967, **21,** 429.
4. For modifications of the Wittig reaction to allow for *cis-* or *trans-*alkene selectivity *see* M. Schlosser and K.F. Christmann, *Angew. Chem. Int. Ed.,* 1966, **5,** 126; M. Schlosser, G. Muller and K.F. Christmann, *Angew. Chem. Int. Ed.,* p 667; W.S. Wadsworth and W.D. Emmons, *J. Am. chem. Soc.,* 1961, **83,** 1733.
5. R.F. NEWTON *et al., J. Chem. Soc., Chem. Commun.,* 1979, 908.
6. P. YATES and R.O. LOUTFY, *Acc. Chem. Res.,* 1975, **8,** 209.
7. D.R. MORTON and N.J. TURRO, *Adv. Photochem.,* 1974, **9,** 198.
8. R.M. MAGID, *Tetrahedron,* 1980, **36,** 1901.

CHAPTER 5

Synthesis of prostaglandins involving conjugate addition to cyclopentenones

Feodor Scheinmann

Department of Chemistry and Applied Chemistry, University of Salford, Lancashire

Introduction

The addition of an organometallic reagent to an α,β-unsaturated carbonyl compound can occur in one or both of two pathways. 1,2-Addition across the carbonyl group results in allylic alcohol formation (*see Figure 5.1*, path ***a***) whereas addition to the entire conjugated system gives the 1,4-adduct and hence the β-substituted carbonyl compound (*see Figure 5.1*, path ***b***). The keto-enol process will lead to the thermodynamically most stable product and therefore steric interactions between the new and resident groups will be largely minimized.

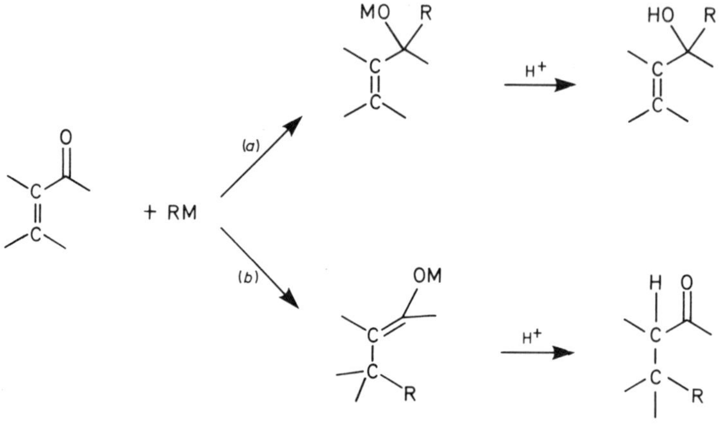

Figure 5.1: Addition of an organometallic reagent to an α,β-unsaturated carbonyl compound

This fact provides us with a simple asymmetric synthesis of prostaglandins, since the stereochemistry of the oxy-substituent at C-4 in the cyclopentenone controls the chirality at C-2 and C-3. Thus, conjugate addition provides the required all-*trans* stereochemistry of the substituents on the cyclopentane ring (*see Figure 5.2*).

By utilizing the reactions of enolate ions, substituents both at C-2 and C-3 may be introduced without isolation of intermediates; thermodynamic

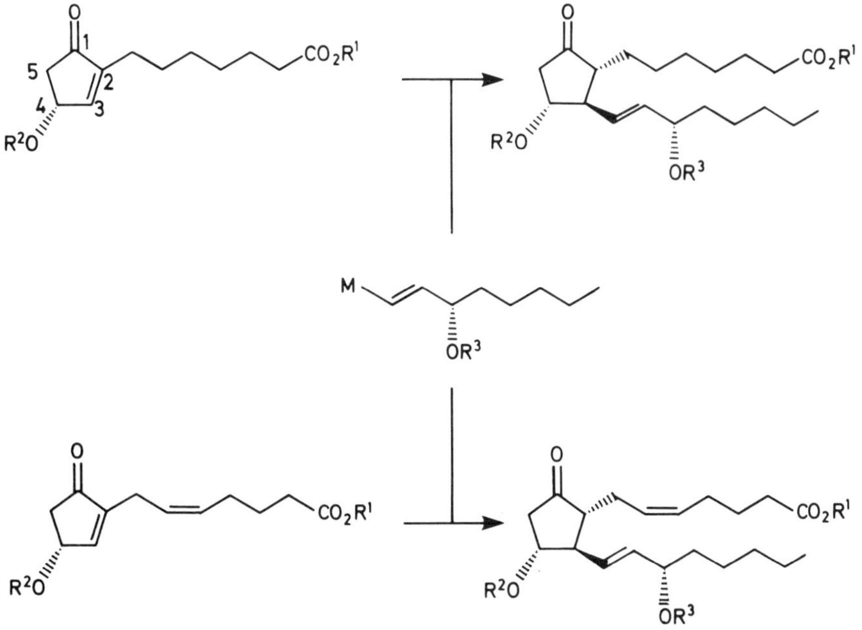

Figure 5.2: Conjugate addition to a 2,4-disubstituted cyclopentenone

control should again favour the *trans*-adduct. This route has provided key prostanoid intermediates which can be converted into prostaglandins and their analogues (*see Figure 5.3*).

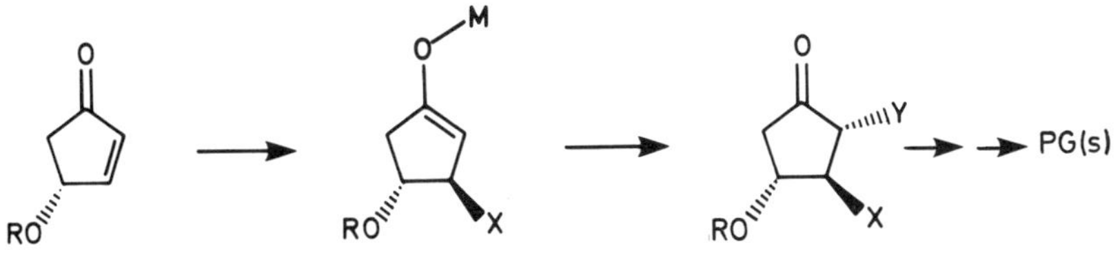

Figure 5.3: Conjugate addition followed by trapping of the enolate with an electrophile

The development of organometallic reagents for conjugate addition reactions

The selective 1,4-addition of Grignard reagents to α,β-unsaturated ketones in the presence of catalytic amounts of copper reagents has been known since 1941. In 1966 House reported that the use of stoichiometric quantities of lithium dialkyl cuprate reagent, $LiCuR_2$, gave exclusively 1,4-adducts. Stoichiometric organocopper reagents generally produce selective conjugate adducts in higher yields and with greater stereoselectivity than copper catalysis. Thus, organocuprates have become the reagents of choice for effecting 1,4-addition to conjugated enones, although the thermal instability of the cuprates require reactions to be carried out between —78 and —20°C.

Several organic derivatives of other Group II metals (Be, Zn, Cd) of the forms RMX, R_2M and R_3MLi undergo conjugate addition in fair to good yields. Metal hydride addition to acetylenes and olefins provide ready access to other organometallic reagents such as alkylboranes, alanes and zirconates which undergo conjugate addition, often aided by the presence of another organometallic reagent.

Synthetic aims

Although the total synthesis of a natural product is often first developed with racemic synthons and reagents to give the racemic modification, it should be the ultimate aim to synthesize the chiral molecule. Ideally, the key synthons should also be readily available as optically pure intermediates with the correct stereochemistry for a convergent synthesis. The approach outlined in *Figure 5.2* fulfils these requirements, since the cyclopentenone and allyl alcohol derivatives each with only one chiral centre lead to PGE_1 (or PGE_2) with four chiral centres.

This chapter reviews the conjugate addition process in *Figure 5.2* and the preparation of the key synthons with emphasis on the routes which lead to the preparation of chiral intermediates. A similar approach will be used to illustrate the synthetic route outlined by *Figure 5.3*, whereby the lower and upper side chains are introduced by conjugate addition followed by trapping of the enolate intermediate with an electrophile.

Conjugate addition to 2,4-disubstituted cyclopentenones
(*see Figure 5.2*)

This approach was successfully pioneered by Sih and co-workers[2,7]. The chiral organocuprate (3) was prepared from 3(*S*)-hydroxy-1-iodo-1-*trans*-octene which was protected as the ethoxy ethyl ether (1) by acid catalyzed reaction with ethyl vinyl ether. Lithiation to give (2) and immediate reaction with tri-n-butyl phosphine copper (I) iodide at −78°C gave the reagent (3), which underwent conjugate addition to the cyclopentenone synthon (4), suitably protected as the tetrahydropyranyl ether ethyl ester. Reaction with the racemic cyclopentenone produced two diastereomers, (5) and (6), which were separated by chromatography after removing the ether protecting group under mild conditions (aqueous acetic acid at 31°C). The hydrolysis of the ester group to give PGE_1 was achieved using baker's yeast in a phosphate buffer, since the β-ketol system is unstable to acidic and basic reagents (*see Figure 5.4*).

The synthesis of (—)-PGE_2 was achieved using two chiral precursors, (7) and (3), and a similar conjugate addition gave yields of 50–60 per cent of (8) (*see Figure 5.5*)[2c].

One of the limitations of this synthesis was that only one vinyl moiety was

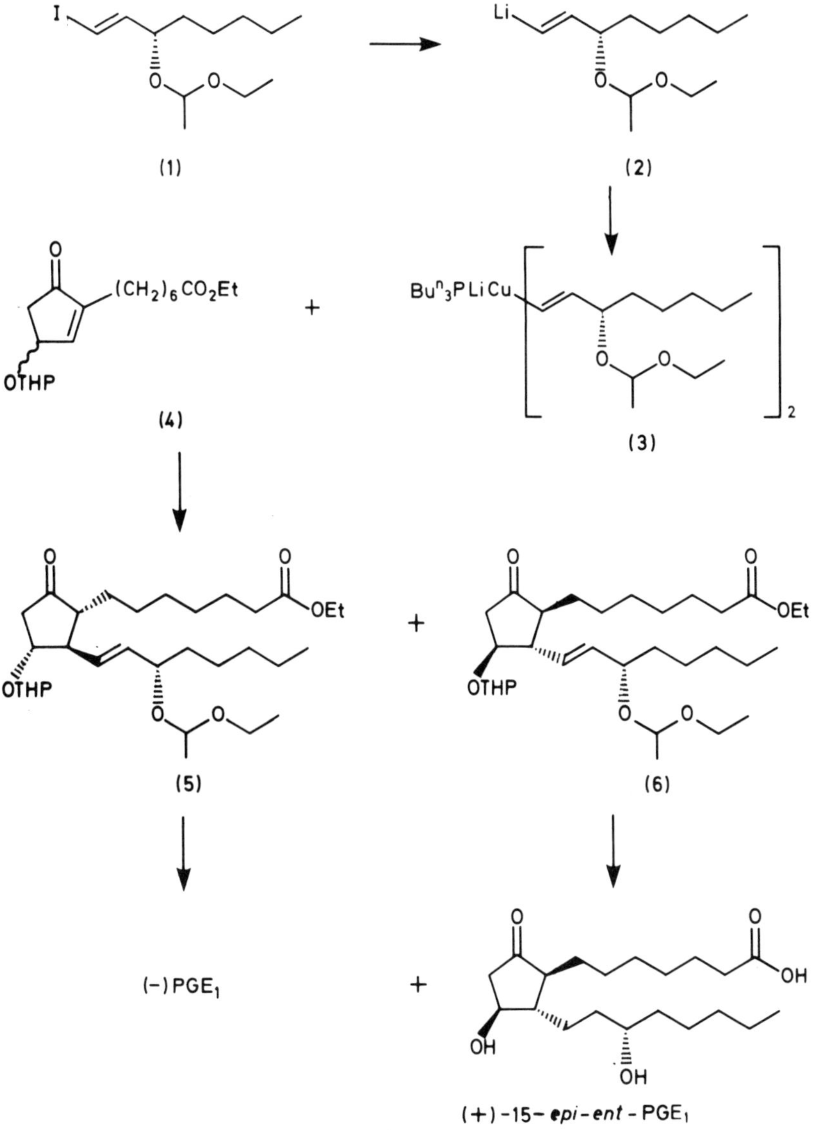

*Figure 5.4: Synthesis of (—)PGE_1 and an isomer (+)-15-*epi-ent-*PGE_1*

transferred from the divinylcuprate reagent. A mixed pentynyl vinylcuprate reagent (9) was prepared (*see Figure 5.6*) whereby only the vinyl group was selectively transferred in the conjugate addition process[3].

Another important modification to the reagent involved the ligand used to complex and solubilize the cuprate. Hexamethylphosphorus triamide has proved to be a successful complexing agent for mixed cuprates[4] and cuprous bromide-dimethyl sulphide complex has also been successfully used with divinylcuprates.

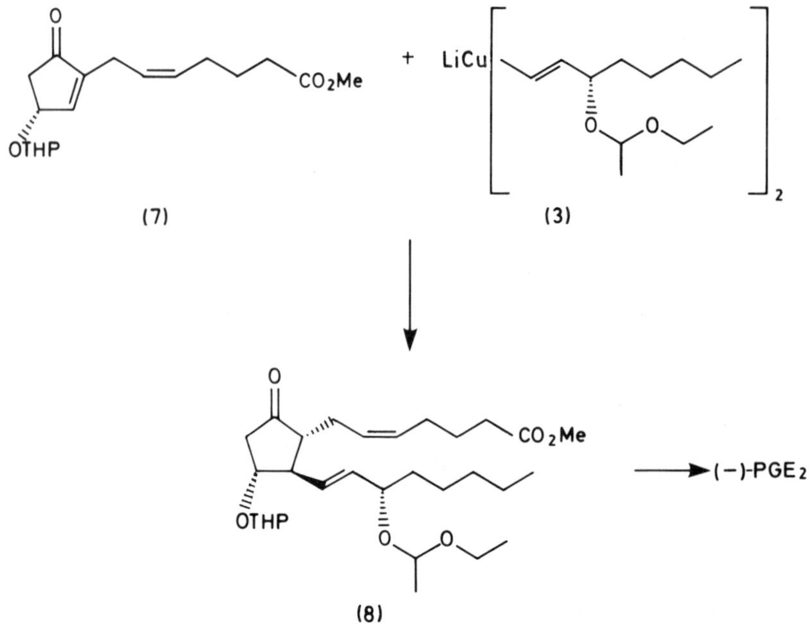

Figure 5.5: Synthesis of (—)PGE$_2$

Success in introducing a *cis* vinyl group as the lower side chain (*see Figure 5.7*) led to alternative methods to prepare the natural prostaglandin[5]. Thus the *cis* allylic alcohol (11) with the wrong chirality at C-15 was transformed into the *trans* allylic alcohol with the correct stereochemistry at C-15 (14). Conversion into the *p*-toluene sulphenate (12) followed by a [2,3] sigmatropic rearrangement gave the sulphoxide (13), which after free rotation reverted to a more stable sulphenate (14), which was converted into PGE$_1$ by treatment with methanolic trimethylphosphite and subsequent hydrolysis.

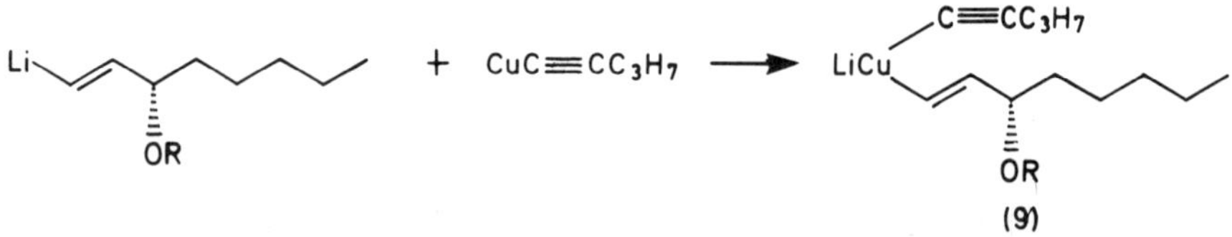

Figure 5.6: Preparation of a hetero cuprate reagent

The use of the copper catalyzed vinyl Grignard reagent is less attractive for conjugate addition reactions because vinyl Grignard reagents are more difficult to prepare and the reaction from the vinylhalide is not totally stereospecific.

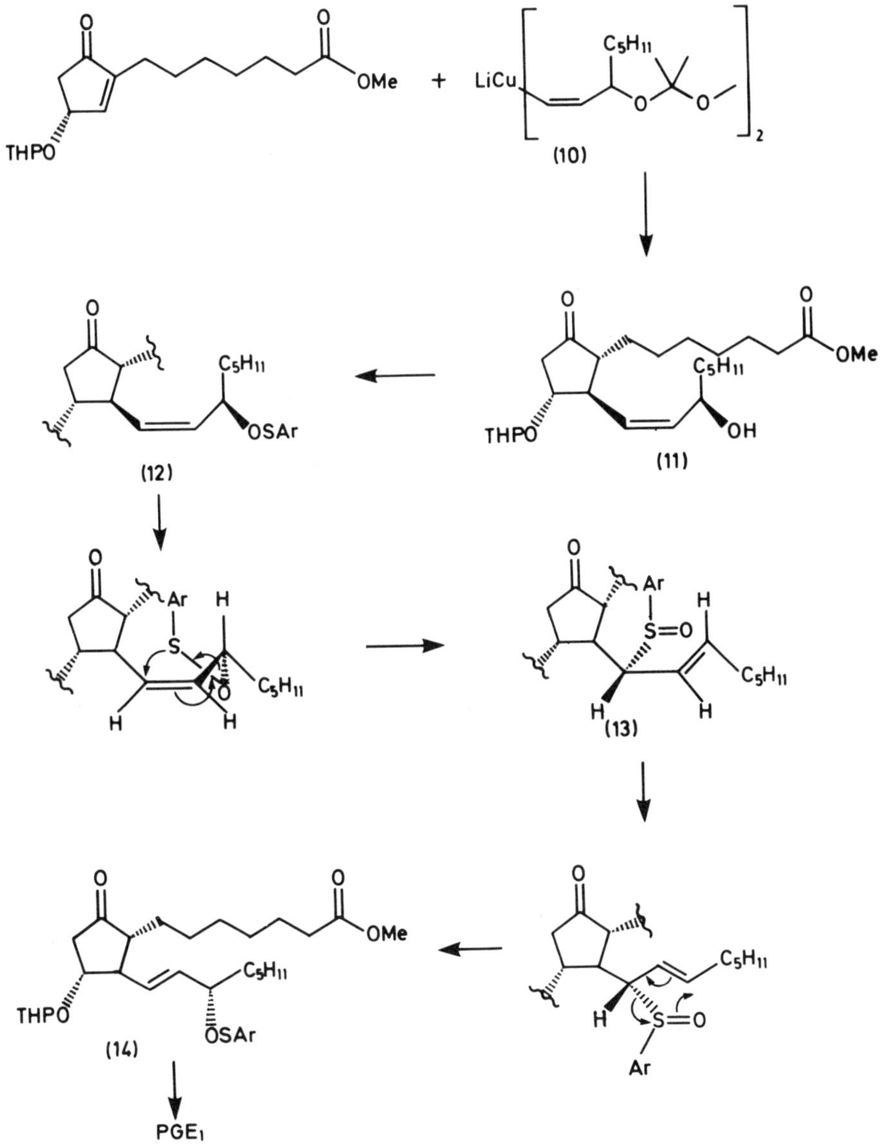

Figure 5.7: Synthesis of PGE_1 using a cis-*vinyl cuprate reagent*

The alanate reagent (16), prepared by the addition of diisobutylaluminium hydride to the propargyl ether (15) followed by addition of methyllithium (or by addition of a trialkylaluminium to the octenyl-lithium) undergoes conjugate addition at room temperature (*see Figure 5.8*), but otherwise the reagent does not have any advantages over the analogous cuprate[6].

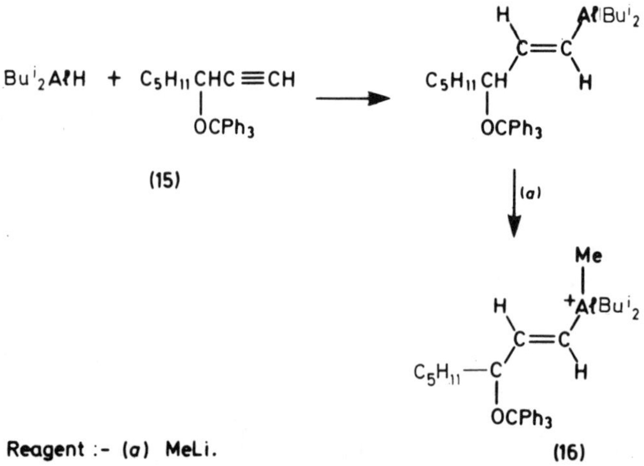

Reagent :- (*a*) MeLi.

Figure 5.8. Preparation of an alanate reagent

Preparation of the (*S*)-1-iodo-3-hydroxyoct-1-ene

Two approaches have been successfully used for the preparation of the chiral octenyl synthon. The first method involved preparation of 1-chloro-oct-1-en-3-one (18) by reaction of acetylene with hexanoyl chloride (17) in the presence of aluminium chloride[3]. Treatment with sodium iodide in acetone gave the corresponding iodo-derivative (19). The optically active alcohol (20) was obtained in about 10 per cent yield by enzymatic reduction with *Penicillium decumbens*[2c]. However, the (*S*)-binaphthol aluminium hydride reagent (21), prepared from optically pure 2,2′-dihydroxy-1,1′-binaphthyl and lithium aluminium hydride in ethanolic tetrahydrofuran, achieves enantioselective reduction in high yield (*see Figure 5.9*)[7].

The alternative route for preparing the chiral side-chain commences from

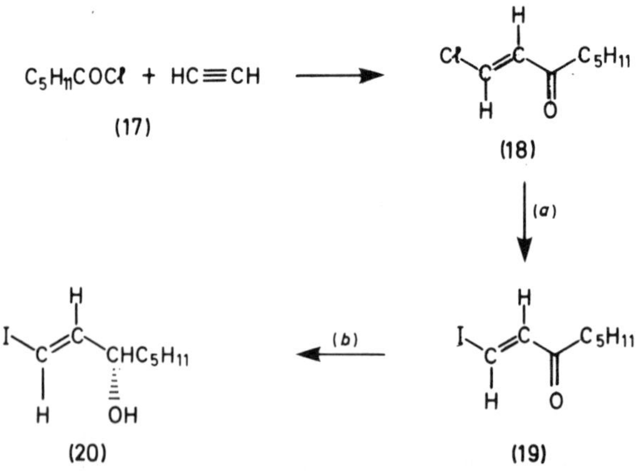

Reagents :- (*a*) NaI, acetone ; (*b*) enzymic reduction or reagent (21).

Figure 5.9: Preparation of (S)-1-iodo-3-hydroxyoct-1-ene

racemic oct-1-yn-3-ol (22). Conversion into the hemiphthalate (23) allowed resolution as the α-phenylethylamine salt (24). Hydrolysis of the hemiphthalate (25) gave the optically pure octyn-3-ol (26)[8]. Addition of

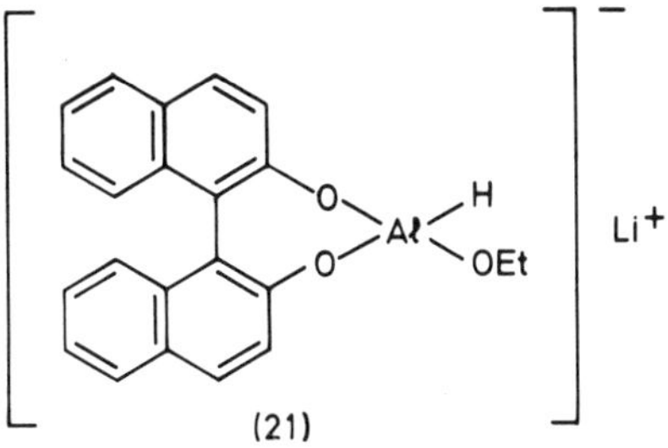

(21)

tributyltin hydride to the triethylsilyl or tetrahydropyranyl ether (27) gave the vinyltin adduct (28), which is converted into 3-(*S*)-hydroxy-1-iodo-1-*trans*-octene with iodine, or directly to the chiral lithio-derivative (29) with butyl lithium (*see Figure 5.10*).

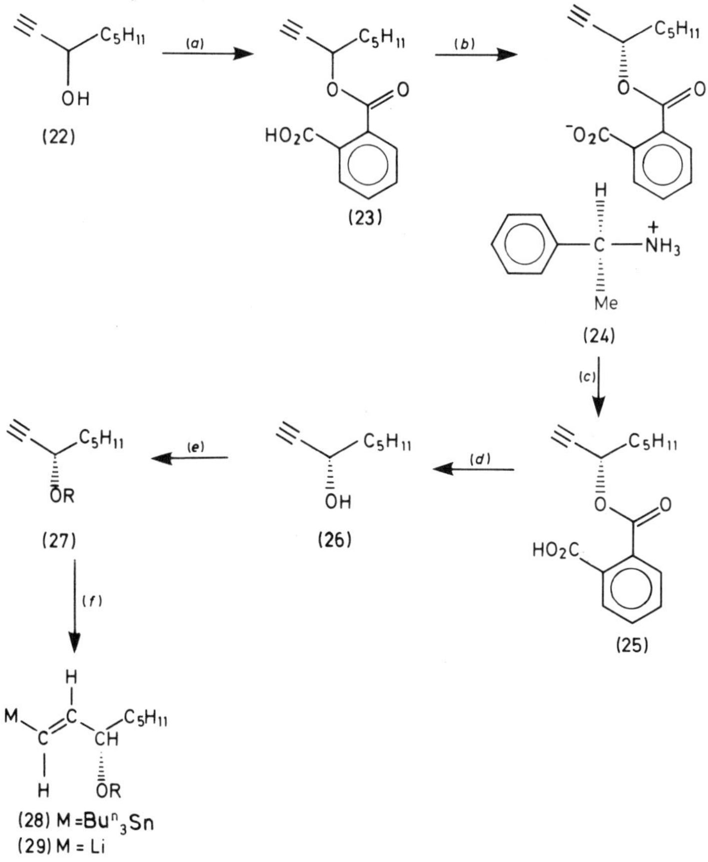

(22) (23) (24) (25) (26) (27)

(28) M = Bu^n_3Sn
(29) M = Li

Reagents:- (*a*) $C_6H_4(CO_2H)_2$; (*b*) (+) − PhCH(Me)NH_2; (*c*) crystallize, then H^+; (*d*) OH^- ; (*e*) protection ; (*f*) $HSnBu^n_3$ then Bu^nLi.

Figure 5.10: Synthesis of 1-metallo-3(S)-alk(silyl)oxyoct-1-ene

Preparation of cyclopentenones used in the conjugate addition reactions

Three approaches have been developed for the preparation of the chiral cyclopentenones shown in *Figure 5.2.* They are based on: (1) resolving the key racemic cyclopentenone prior to conjugate addition; (2) incorporation of an enantiospecific reaction in the synthesis; and (3) using a chiral starting material with the correct configuration of the hydroxyl at C-4 (C-11 prostaglandin numbering).

There are now a number of syntheses for preparing the racemic α-alkylated cyclopentenones and chemists at the Searle laboratories have demonstrated that 2-(6-methoxycarbonylhexyl)-4-hydroxycyclopent-2-en-1-one may be resolved after oxime formation with (*R*)-2-aminooxy-4-methylvaleric acid (30)[9]. The diastereomeric mixture of oximes was separated by

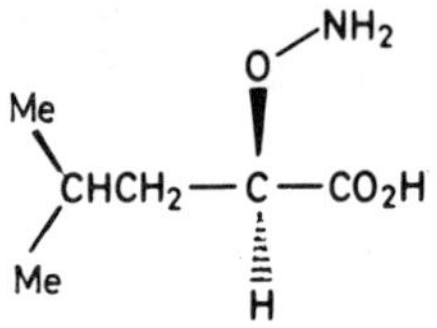

(30)

chromatography and the required ketone was regenerated using titanium trichloride in aqueous tetrahydrofuran buffered with ammonium acetate (*see Figure 5.11*).

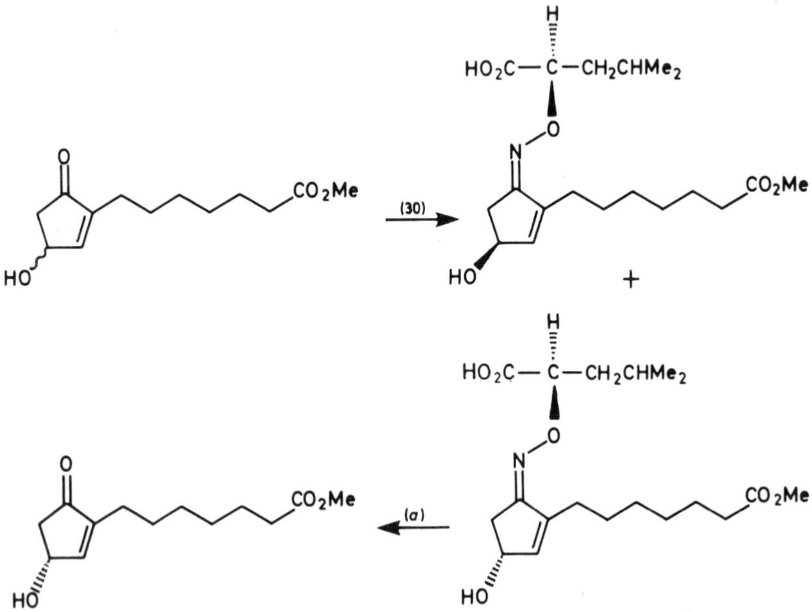

Reagents: (*a*) $TiCl_3$, NH_4OAc

Figure 5.11: Resolution of 2-(6-methoxycarbonylhexyl)-4-hydroxycyclopent-2-en-1-one

Sih and his co-workers used decanoic acid derivatives (31) and (33) as the key synthons for the preparation of the required cyclopentenones. Thus, 9-oxodecanoic acid (31) was converted into the triketone (32) by reaction with dimethyl oxalate in the presence of potassium t-butoxide. The triketone (34) required for the preparation of PGE_2 was synthesized in a similar way (*see Figure 5.12*)[2].

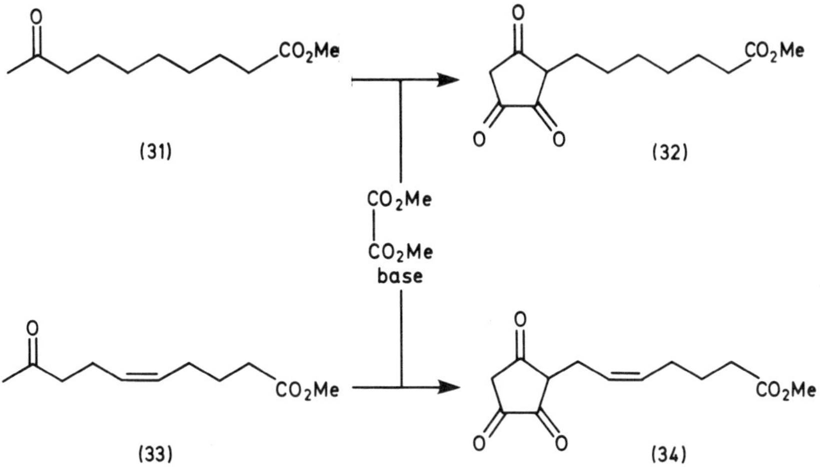

Figure 5.12: The synthesis of methoxycarbonylhex(en)ylcyclopentanetriones

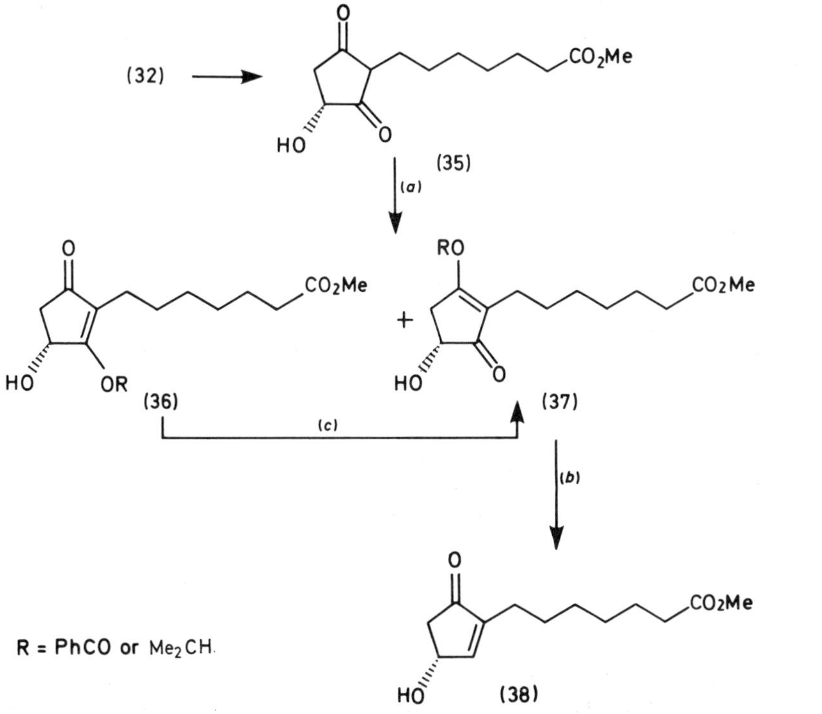

R = PhCO or Me_2CH

Reagents :- (*a*) RX, base ; (*b*) $LiAl(OCH_2CH_2OMe)_2H_2$; (*c*) HCl.

Figure 5.13: Conversion of a cyclopentanetrione into a PGE_1 precursor

Enzymatic reduction of (32) using *Dipodascus uninucleatus* gave the *R*-alcohol (35). This asymmetric reduction has also been achieved chemically for (32) in about 54 per cent optical purity using lithium aluminium hydride partly decomposed by (—)-*N*-methylephedrine. Conversion into the enol benzoate or isopropyl enol ether gave a mixture, (36) and (37), which was converted into the sterically less crowded enolate at C-9 (37) in the presence of a trace of acid. Reduction of the carbonyl followed by acid-catalysed allylic rearrangement afforded the desired chiral cyclopentenone (38) (*see Figure 5.13*). A similar sequence of reactions were carried out to prepare the chiral cyclopentenone intermediate (39) for conversion into PGE_2.

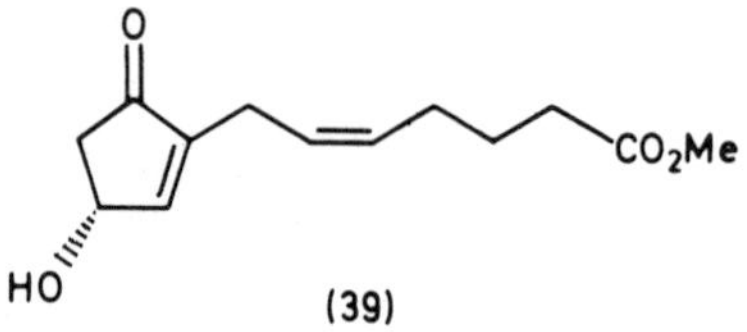

O

CO_2Me

HO

(39)

Another approach to the cyclopentenone synthon involves reaction of lithium cyclopentadienide with ethyl 7-bromoheptanoate to give a mixture of alkylated cyclopentadiene isomers, for example (40). Reaction with singlet oxygen, generated by the interaction of sodium hypochlorite and hydrogen peroxide in methanol at $-10°C$, gave by the intermediacy of the endoperoxide (41) a 1:4 mixture of hydroxycyclopentenones (42) and (43) which was readily separated by chromatrography. To obtain a better yield of the desired cyclopentenone (42), the mixture (42) and (43) was oxidized with chromium trioxide (Jones reagent) to the diketone (44) which, when reduced back with aluminium isopropoxide, gave the hydroxycyclopentenones (42) and (43) in a ratio of 1:2 (*see Figure 5.14*)[2b].

Another approach starts from the chiral cyclopentene lactone (45)[10] which was hydroxylated with osmium tetroxide and aqueous sodium chlorate (*see Figure 5.15*). Protection of the diol (46) as the acetone ketal (47) and reduction of the lactone to the lactol with diisobutylaluminium hydride, followed by a Wittig olefination with the ylide derived from triphenylphosphoniopentanoic acid, gave the α-side chain. Methyl ester formation and oxidation of the cyclopentanol (48) with chromium trioxide-pyridine complex gave the cyclopentanone (49). The required chiral cyclopentenone (50) was obtained by hydrolysis of the ketal and dehydration in a two phase system containing oxalic acid, sodium oxalate and chloroform.

A novel approach to the racemic cyclopentenone was developed by Floyd[11]. The retrosynthetic analysis is shown in *Figure 5.16*. The cyclopentenolone isomerization (52→51) can occur under various conditions as illustrated in *Figure 5.17*. The conversion from the 2,5-dihydro-2,5-dimethoxyfuran was achieved in 'one pot' using a phosphate buffer at pH 6 in aqueous dioxan at 92°C for the ketal hydrolysis (54→53) and aldol cyclization (53→52), followed by acidification to a concentration of 0.5 molar

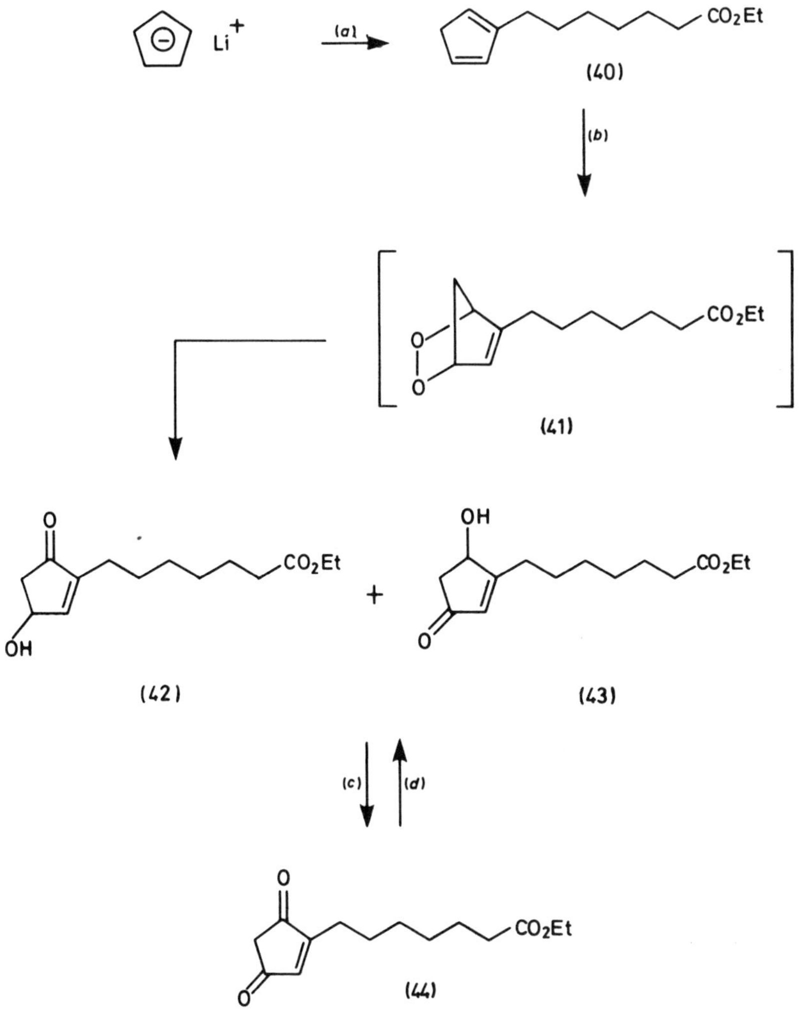

Reagents :- (*a*) $BrCH_2(CH_2)_5CO_2Et$; (*b*) $NaOCl$, H_2O_2, MeOH ; (*c*) CrO_3, H^+;
(*d*) $Al(OCHMe_2)_3$

Figure 5.14: Synthesis of PG precursors from a cyclopentadiene derivative using singlet oxygen

sulphuric acid for the cyclopentanolone isomerization (52→51). The dihydro dimethoxyfuran (54) was easily synthesized by standard methods as shown in *Figure 5.18.*

Another general approach involves preparation of the 2-alkylated cyclopentenone (56) (*see Figure 5.19*) followed by hydroxylation at C-4. The allylic hydroxylation can be achieved enzymatically with *Aspergillus niger*[12] or alternatively by allylic bromination followed by hydrolysis with aqueous silver salts[13].

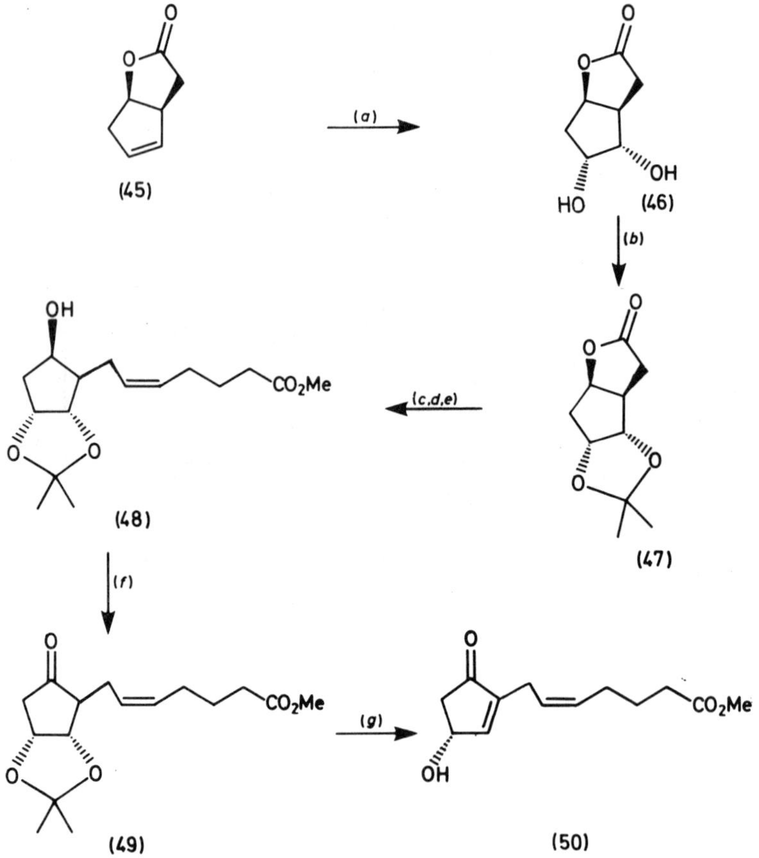

(45) (46) (47) (48) (49) (50)

Reagents :- (a) OsO_4, $NaClO_3$; (b) Me_2CO , H^+ ; (c) $Bu^i{}_2AlH$; (d) $Ph_3PCH(CH_2)_3CO_2H$; (e) CH_2N_2 ; (f) CrO_3 , pyridine ; (g) $(CO_2H)_2$, NaOH, $CHCl_3$.

Figure 5.15: Synthesis of a PGE$_2$ precursor from 2-oxabicyclo[3.3.0]oct-6-en-3-one

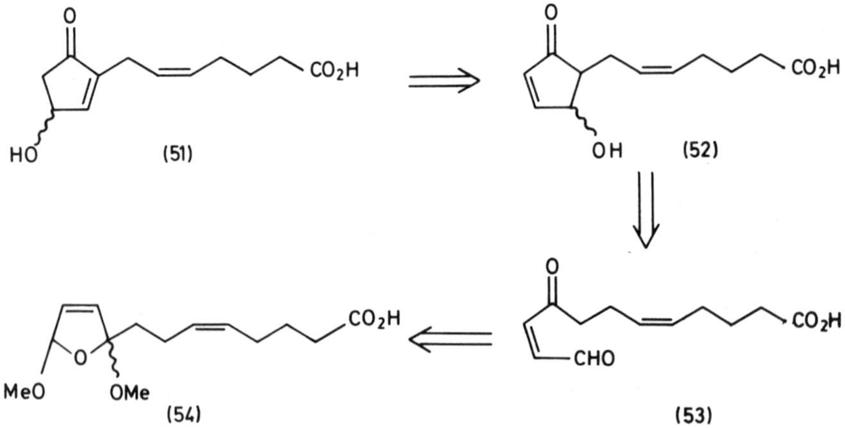

(51) (52) (53) (54)

Figure 5.16. Retrosynthetic analysis of the route to enone (51).

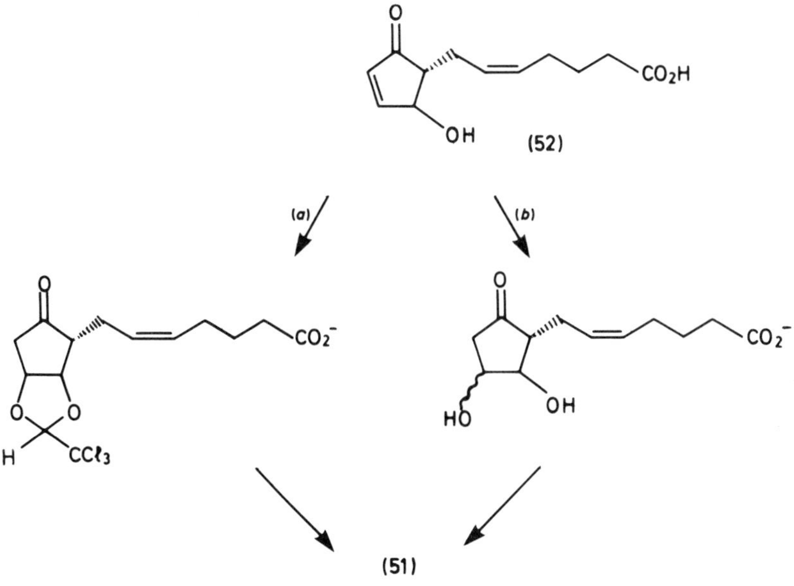

(52)

(51)

Reagents: (a), Et_3N, CCl_3CHO; (b), CO_3^{2-}, pH 10.

Figure 5.17: Isomerization of a cyclopentenolone

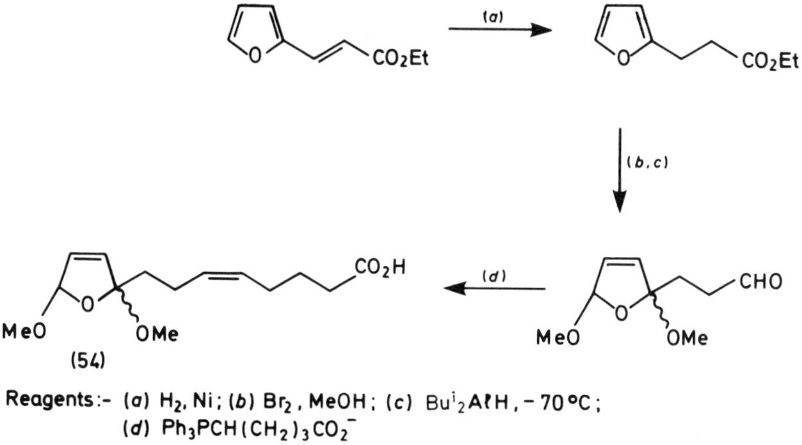

(54)

Reagents:- (a) H_2, Ni; (b) Br_2, MeOH; (c) $Bu^i{}_2AlH$, − 70 °C;
(d) $Ph_3PCH(CH_2)_3CO_2^-$

Figure 5.18: Synthesis of the dimethoxydihydrofuran (54)

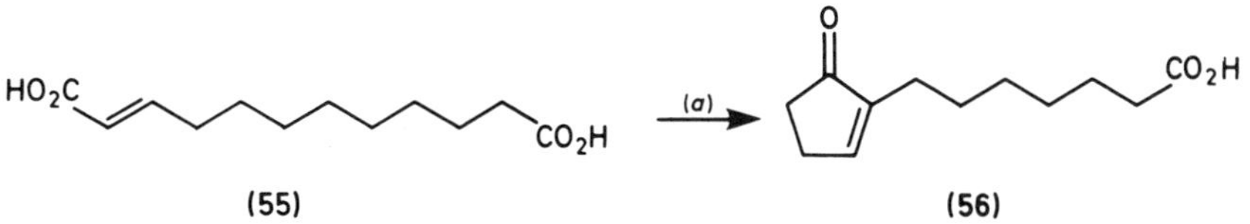

(55) (56)

Reagent: (a) polyphosphoric acid

Figure 5.19: Preparation of 2-(carboxyhexyl)cyclopent-2-enone

Since 11-deoxyprostaglandins are themselves of pharmacological interest, a number of syntheses of the cyclopentenone (56) have been developed. Cyclization of traumatic acid (55) with polyphosphoric acid gives the required cyclopentenone (56) in one step (*see Figure 5.19*)[14]. For large quantities of the cyclopentenone (56) from cheap starting materials, an enamine synthesis from cyclopentanone has been utilized[15]. The total syntheses of PGD_1 (*see Figure 5.20*) and TXB_1 illustrate this approach and the value of carefully selected protecting groups[13]. Cyclopentanone was converted into the morpholine enamine (57) and reaction with 7-hydroxyheptanal gave the exocyclic cyclopentenone (58), which was isomerized to (59) by hydrochloric acid in butanol at 90°C. Oxidation with Jones reagent followed by methylation gave the required methyl ester (60) in 25 per cent yield from cyclopentanone. Allylic bromination with *N*-bromosuccinimide followed by hydrolysis with aqueous silver perchlorate gave the 4-hydroxycyclopentenone (61), which was separated from its isomer (62) by

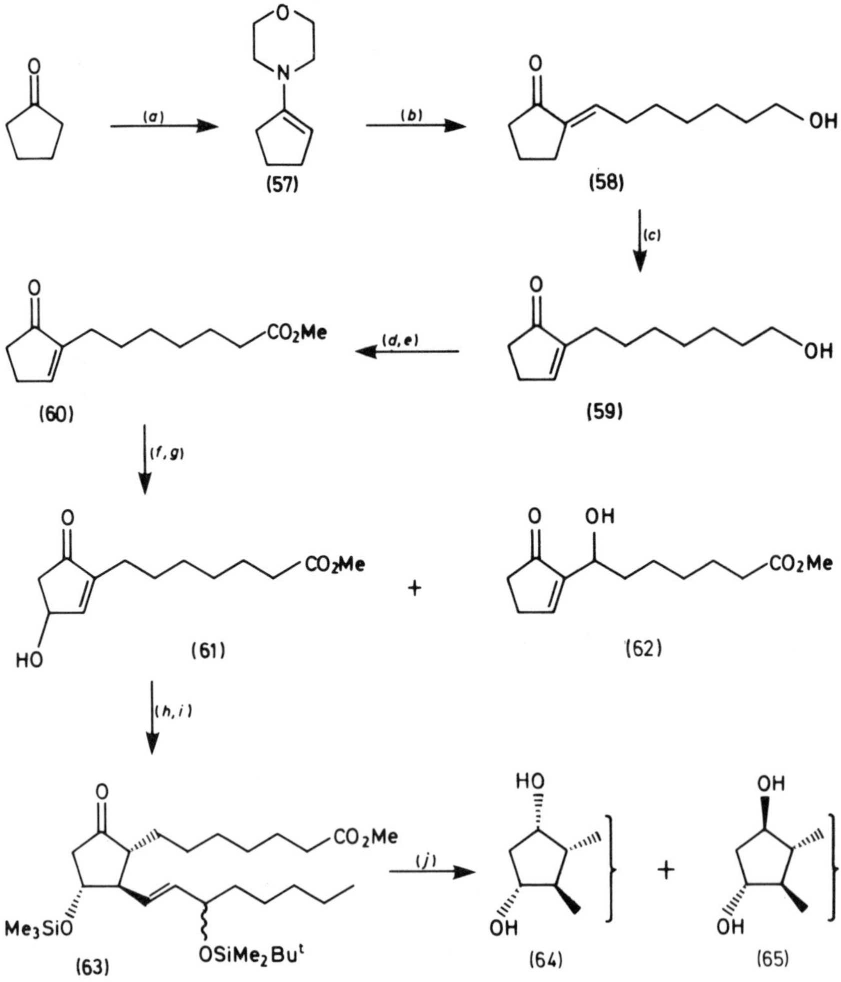

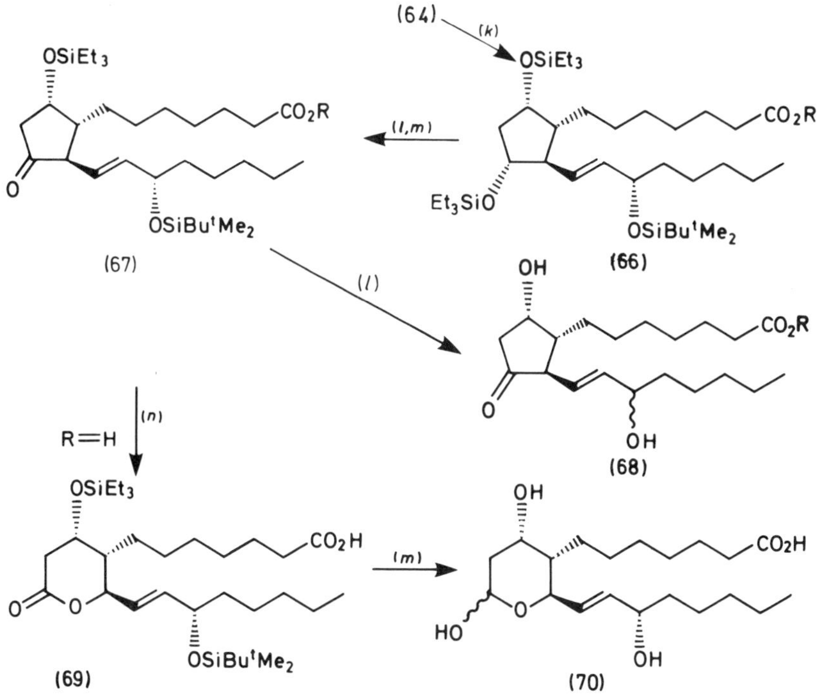

Reagents:- (*a*) morpholine (O NH), H_2O; (*b*) $HOCH_2(CH_2)_5CHO$; (*c*) H^+; (*d*) CrO_3;
(*e*) CH_2N_2; (*f*) NBS,*hν*; (*g*) $AgClO_4$, H_2O; (*h*) Me_3SiCl base;
(*i*) LiCuR(CH=CH)CH(OSiBu^{t}Me$_2$) C_5H_{11}; (*j*) H^+ brief treatment;
(*k*) Et_3SiCl base; (*l*) $MeCO_2H$, H_2O; (*m*) pyridinium chlorochromate;
(*n*) peracid

Figure 5.20: Conjugate addition reaction leading to prostaglandin D_1 and thromboxane B_1

chromatography. For the synthesis of PGD_1 it was necessary to use different protecting groups for the hydroxyls in the rings and the side chain, so that the oxy function at C-15 would remain unchanged while those in the ring were being modified. The 4-hydroxyl group in the cyclopentenone (61) was therefore protected as the labile trimethylsilyl ether, and the 1-iodo-1-(*E*)-octenol as the more stable t-butyldimethylsilyl ether. The conjugate addition reaction with the mixed cuprate (9) gave the racemic PGE_1 derivative (63), which was reduced with sodium borohydride to a 3:1 mixture of $PGF_{1\alpha}$ (64) and $PGF_{1\beta}$ (65) 15-t-butyldimethylsilyl ether methyl esters. Alkaline hydrolysis of the $PGF_{1\alpha}$ derivative gave the acid. Both the acid and its methyl ester form the 9,11-bistriethylsilyl ether derivative (66) which can be selectively hydrolyzed, at the sterically less hindered C-11 position, prior to or on oxidation with pyridinium chlorochromate to give the 11-oxo derivative (67). More vigorous hydrolysis with aqueous acetic acid in tetrahydrofuran gave (±)-PGD_1 and (±)-15-epi-PGD_1 (68) (*see Figure 5.20*). A Baeyer-Villiger oxidation of the 11-oxo group (67) followed by reduction of the lactone (69) with diisobutylaluminium hydride provides an approach to TXB_1 (70).

An elegant method for the preparation of the chiral cyclopentenone (71) utilizes D-glyceraldehyde[16]. In a retroanalysis, one may envisage that the acyl anion equivalent (73) forms the cyclopentenone (71) by a nucleophilic displacement and an aldol reaction with the 3-tosylate of D-glyceraldehyde (72) (*see Figure 5.21*).

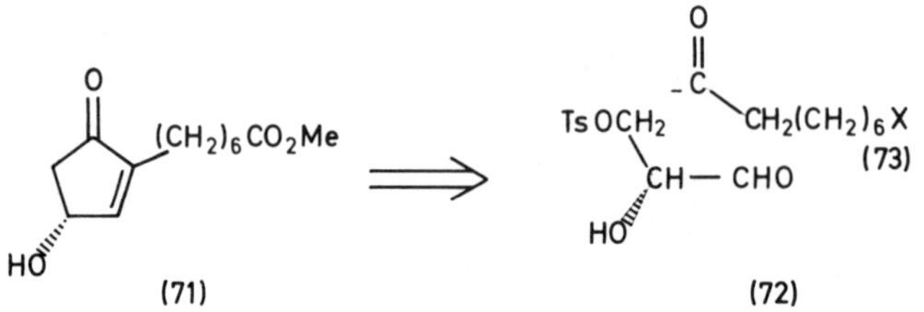

Figure 5.21: Retrosynthetic analysis of the production of a 4-hydroxycyclopent-2-enone from a three-carbon unit derived from D-glyceraldehyde

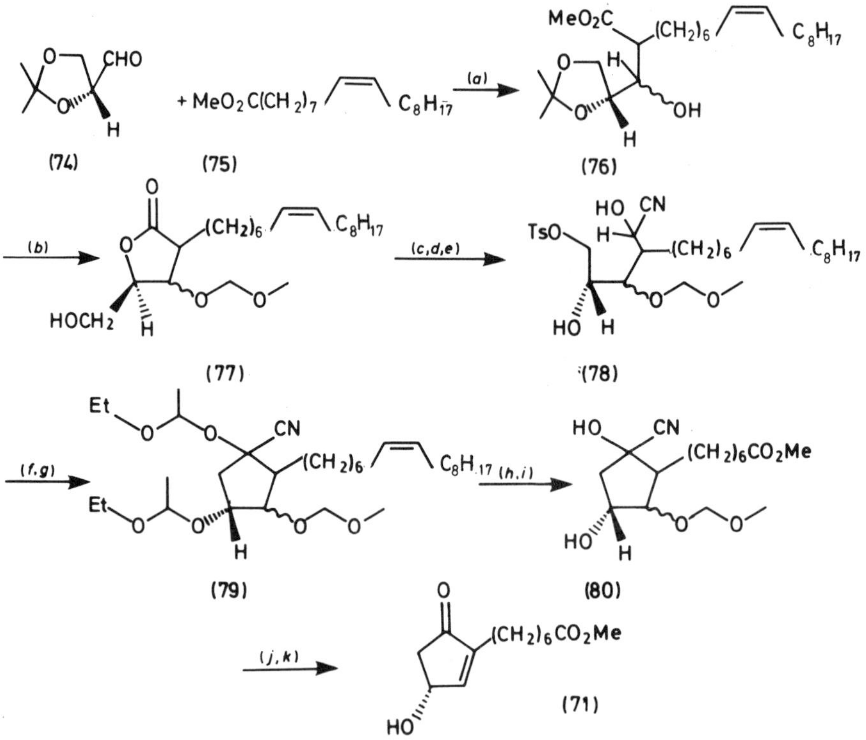

Reagents:- (*a*) Pr_2^iNLi; (*b*) $ClCH_2OMe$; (*c*) TsCl; (*d*) Bu^i_2AlH; (*e*) HCN, EtOH, NH_4OH; (*f*) $CH_2{:}CHOEt$; (*g*) $NaNR_2$; (*h*) $NaIO_4$, $KMnO_4$, (*i*) CH_2N_2; (*j*) NaOH; (*k*) HCl.

Figure 5.22: Synthesis of PGE_2 precursor (71) from D-glyceraldehyde

Despite the simplicity of the concept, the synthesis is lengthy as shown in *Figure 5.22*. Isopropylidene D-glyceraldehyde (74) and methyl oleate (75) were condensed to give the aldol (76). Protection of the new hydroxyl group as the methoxymethyl ether and removal of the isopropylidine moiety led to the formation of the γ-lactone (77). The primary alcohol group was converted into the tosylate and the lactone was converted into the cyanohydrin (78) by reduction with diisobutylaluminium hydride followed by treatment with hydrogen cyanide. The acyl anion equivalent from the ethoxyethyl ether of (78) was formed in the presence of a sodium amide derivative (sodium hexamethyldisilazane) and gave the cyclopentane (79). Cleavage of the double bond with sodium periodate and potassium permanganate followed by removal of the protecting groups and esterification gave the cyanohydrin ester (80). Hydrolysis and base catalyzed elimination gave the required cyclopentenone (71).

Prostaglandin synthesis by conjugate addition and enolate trapping

Probably the shortest approach to prostaglandins involves the conjugate addition of the lower side chain to a 4-alkoxycyclopent-2-enone (81) followed by trapping the enolate with either the whole of the α-side chain or a function which is readily converted into the α-side chain (83).

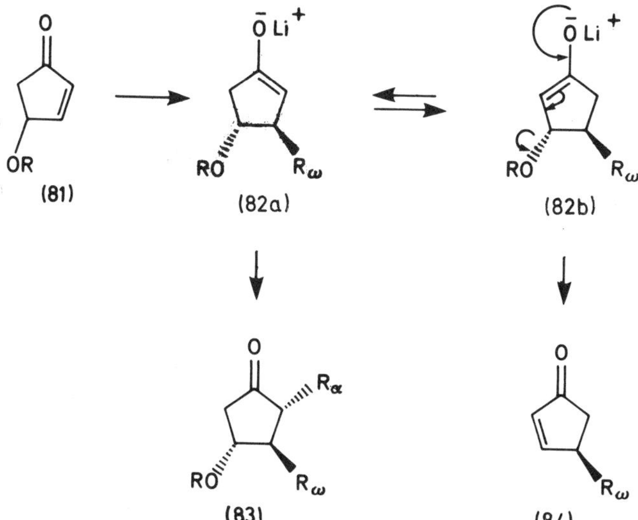

Figure 5.23: The concept of conjugate addition followed by enolate trapping

The reactivity of the electrophile for trapping the enolate is critical for success, otherwise equilibration (82a, 82b) and elimination to give the cyclopentenone (84) may predominate (*see Figure 5.23*).

Thus, while this direct approach was successful for the synthesis of 11-deoxyprostaglandins (e.g. (85)), from cyclopentenone (*see Figure 5.24*)[17] and for the 7-oxoprostaglandin E_1 (86) from 4-t-butyldimethylsiloxycyclopent-2-enone (*see Figure 5.25*)[18], the synthesis of the E-prostaglandins required prior formation of an α-side chain intermediate to rapidly trap the enolate ion.

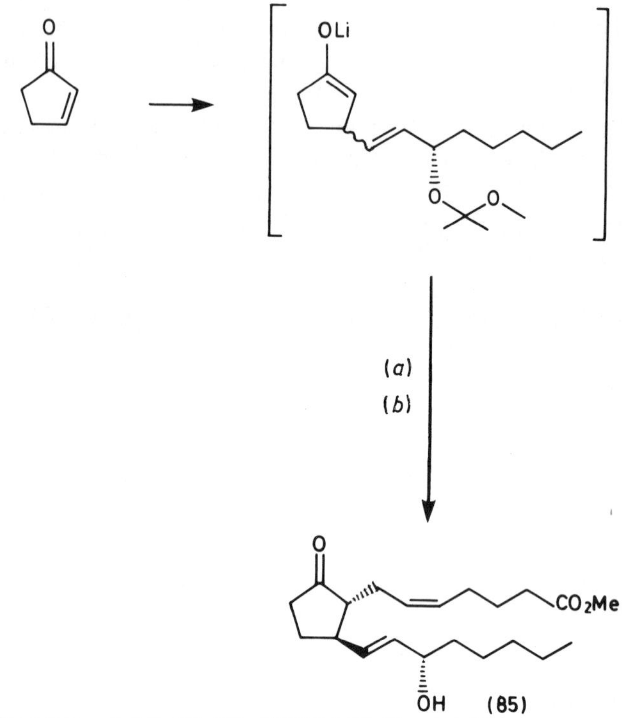

(*a*)
(*b*)

(85)

Reagents:- (*a*) $BrCH_2CH:CH(CH_2)_3CO_2Me$; (*b*) H^+.

Figure 5.24: Synthesis of 11-deoxy-PGE$_2$ derivative

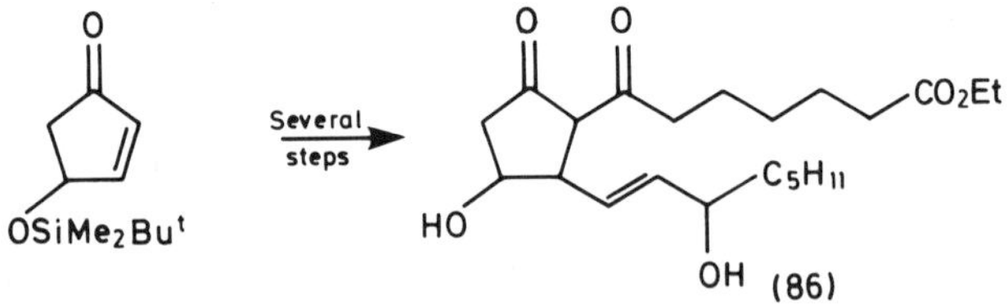

Several steps

(86)

Figure 5.25: Outline of the synthesis of the 7-oxo-PGE$_1$ derivative (86)

The synthesis by Stork and Isobe[19] illustrates that the trapping of the kinetic enol is achieved with formaldehyde which then provides the necessary functionality for conversion into the α-side chain. 4-Cumyloxy-2-cyclopentenone (87) was prepared in 48 per cent yield from cyclopentadiene: 1,4-addition with the chiral cuprate (88) gave the lithium enolate (89).

Trapping with formaldehyde at −78°C gave the hydroxymethylcyclopentanone (90) and its diastereoisomer (91) in a ratio of 1.3:1. The synthesis was concluded by another conjugate addition reaction on the methylenecyclopentanone (92) with the divinylcuprate reagent (93) to give the cyclopentanone (94). Hydrolysis of the ethoxy ethyl protecting group and oxidation with chromium trioxide gave the carboxylic acid (95), which was converted into $PGF_{2\alpha}$ by reduction to the 9-α-hydroxy derivative (96), followed by ether cleavage with sodium or lithium in liquid ammonia (*see Figure 5.26*).

The importance of the α-methylenecyclopentanone, for example (92), in prostaglandin synthesis has led to various syntheses of this intermediate. An interesting development has been the use of alkenylzirconium species for conjugate addition[20]. The reagent is readily prepared by hydrozirconation of an acetylene using $Cp_2Zr.HCl$ [chlorobis(η-cyclopentadienyl) hydridozirconium], which results in a stereospecific *cis*-addition. Transfer of the alkenyl group from the zirconium reagent in a conjugate addition process

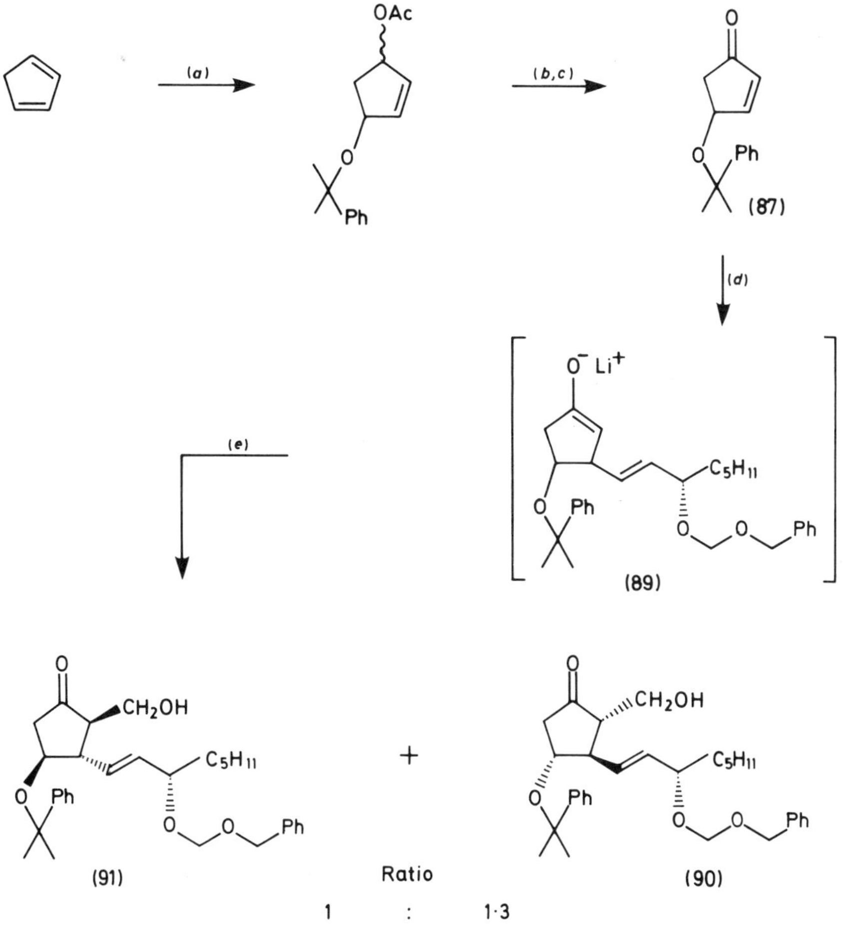

(a) (b,c) (87) (d) (89) (e) (91) (90)

Ratio

1 : 1·3

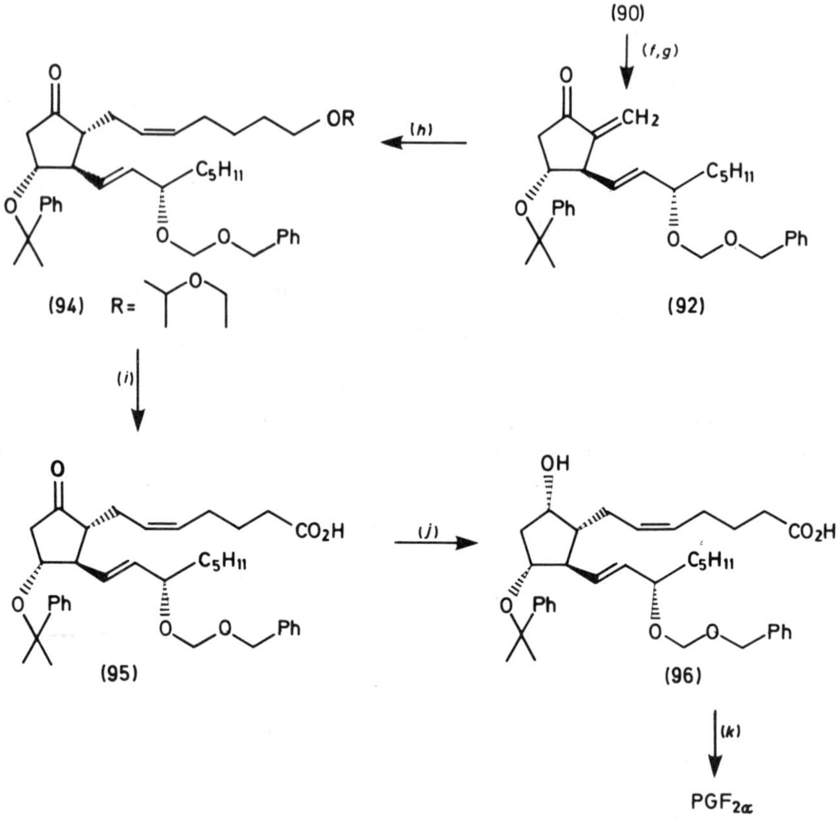

Reagents:- (a) PhC(Me)$_2$OOH then $FeSO_4$, Cu(OAc)$_2$, HOAc; (b) KOH; (c) CrO_3; (d) (88); (e) HCHO, Et_2O, −78 °C; (f) MsCl, C_5H_5N; (g) Pr^{i}NEt; (h) (93); (i) H^+, CrO_3; (j) LiBu$^i_3$BH$_3$; (k) Li, NH_3.

Figure 5.26: Synthesis of $PGF_{2\alpha}$ by Stork and Isobe

was catalyzed by a 1:1 ratio of nickel (II) 2,4-pentanedionate [Ni(AcAc)$_2$] and diisobutylaluminium hydride. Without use of the catalyst, the reaction proceeds only slowly and in low yield. The catalyst, Ni(AcAc)$_2$ activated by reduction, is probably a reduced nickel species generated by transfer of alkenyl from zirconium to nickel, and results in the conversion of the cyclopentenone (87) into the adduct (90) at 0°C in 70 per cent yield.

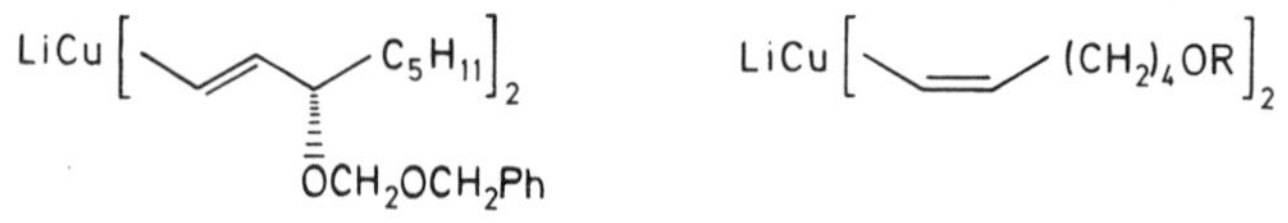

(88) (93)

References

1. G.H. POSNER, *Org. React.*, 1972, **19**, 1.
2. (a) C.J. SIH *et al., J. Am. chem. Soc.*, 1972, **94**, 3643; (b) *idem., J. Am. chem. Soc.*, 1975, **97**, 857; (c) *J. Am. chem. Soc.*, 1975, **97**, 865.
3. E.J. COREY and D.J. BEAMES, *J. Am. chem. Soc.*, 1972, **94**, 7210.
4. H.C. ARNDT *et al., Prostaglandins,* 1974, **7**, 387.
5. A. KLUGE, K.G. UNTCH and J.H. FRIED, *J. Am. chem. Soc.*, 1972, **94**, 9256; J.G. MILLER *et al., J. Am. chem. Soc.*, 1974, **96**, 6774.
6. K.F. BERNADY *et al., J. org. Chem.*, 1979, **44**, 1438.
7. R. NOYORI, I. TOMINO and M. NISHIZAWA, *J. Am. chem. Soc.*, 1979, **101**, 5843.
8. J. FRIED *et al., Ann. N.Y. Acad. Sci.*, 1971, **180**, 39.
9. R. PAPPO, P. COLLINS and C. JUNG, *Tetrahedron Lett.*, 1973, 943.
10. L. GRUBER *et al., Tetrahedron Lett.*, 1974, 3729.
11. M.B. FLOYD, in *Chemistry, Biochemistry and Pharmacological Activity of Prostanoids,* Eds. S.M. Roberts and F. Scheinmann, Pergamon Press, 1979, p 161.
12. S. KUROZUMI, T. TORU and S. ISHIMOTO, *Tetrahedron Letts.*, 1973, 4959.
13. T.W. HART, D.A. METCALFE and F. SCHEINMANN in *ref 11*, p 75; *J. Chem. Soc. Chem. Commun.*, 1979, 156.
14. A.S.C.P. RAO, V.R. NAYAK and S. DEV., *Synthesis,* 1975, 608.
15. T.S. BURTON *et al., J.C.S. Perkin 1,* 1976, 2550.
16. G. STORK and T. TAKAHASHI, *J. Am. chem. Soc.*, 1977, **99**, 1275.
17. J.W. PATTERSON and J.H. FRIED, *J. org. Chem.*, 1974, **39**, 2506.
18. T. TANAKA *et al., Tetrahedron Lett.*, 1975, 1535.
19. G. STORK and M. ISOBE, *J. Am. chem. Soc.*, 1975, **97**, 6260.
20. J. SCHWARTZ, M.L. LOOTS and H. KOSUGI, *J. Am. chem. Soc.*, 1980, **102**, 1333.

General References

J.S. BINDRA and R. BINDRA, *Prostaglandin Synthesis*, Academic Press (New York), 1977, p 99.

A. MITRA, *The Synthesis of Prostaglandins,* John Wiley & Sons (New York), 1977, p 247 and 267.

S.M. ROBERTS and F. SCHEINMANN, *New Synthetic Routes to Prostaglandins and Thromboxanes,* Academic Press (London), 1982.

CHAPTER 6

Chemical interconversions of prostaglandins: synthesis of prostaglandins G_2, H_2, and I_2

Roger F. Newton
Chemical Research Department, Glaxo Group Research, Ware, Hertfordshire
and
Stanley M. Roberts
Chemical Research Department, Glaxo Group Research, Greenford, Middlesex

Introduction

The chemical interconversion of prostaglandins D, E and F and the interconversion of prostaglandins A, B, C and E are dealt with briefly in this chapter[1]. Methods for converting prostaglandins of the 2-series into the corresponding compounds in the 1-series are also outlined[1]. The more important interconversions, namely the production of prostaglandins G_2, H_2, and I_2 from prostaglandin $F_{2\alpha}$, are described in more detail in the latter part of this chapter.

Chemical interconversions of prostaglandins D, E and F

Prostaglandin E_2 was reduced to prostaglandin $F_{2\alpha}$ stereo-specifically using a bulky trialkylborohydride reducing reagent (*see Figure 6.1*). The bulky reagent determines that delivery of the hydride ion takes place from the less-crowded β-face of the five-membered ring. Similarly, borohydride reagents reduced prostaglandin D_2 to $PGF_{2\alpha}$.

The preparation of PGE_2 from $PGF_{2\alpha}$ required the selective protection of the hydroxyl groups at C-11 and C-15. This was achieved in a straightforward fashion employing the methyl ester and through formation of the corresponding 11,15-bis(trimethylsilyl)prostaglandin (1): the hydroxyl group at C-9 did not react with the silylating reagent since it was shielded by the vicinal C_7 side-chain. Oxidation of the secondary alcohol moiety in (1) followed by deprotection afforded PGE_2.

The synthesis of prostaglandin D_2 from $PGF_{2\alpha}$ also takes advantage of the sterically hindered situation of the hydroxyl group at C-9. A cyclic boronate spanning the oxygen atoms at C-9 and C-11 was formed and the free hydroxyl group at C-15 was protected as the tetrahydropyranyl derivative to give (2). The boronate ester was removed using peroxide to give

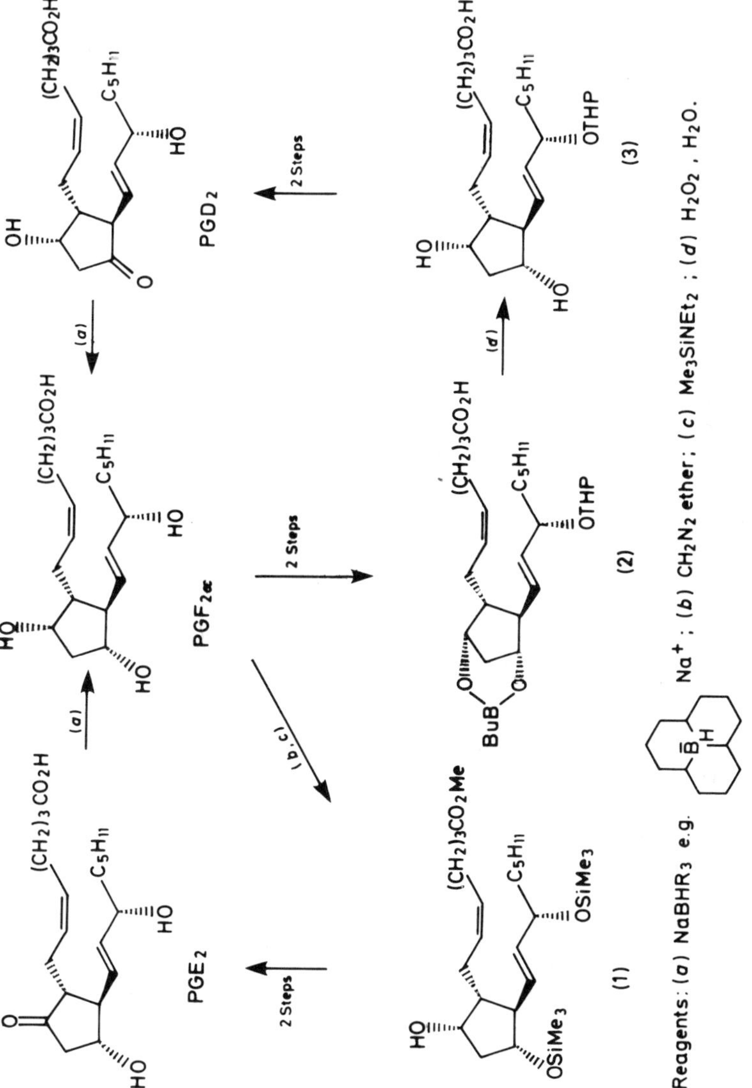

Figure 6.1: Interconversion of prostaglandins D_2, E_2 and $F_{2\alpha}$

(3). The diol (3) was then selectively oxidized using Jones reagent, the more accessible hydroxyl group at C-11 being oxidized preferentially. Removal of the tetrahydropyranyl protecting group gave PGD_2 in *ca.* 20 per cent yield from $PGF_{2\alpha}$.

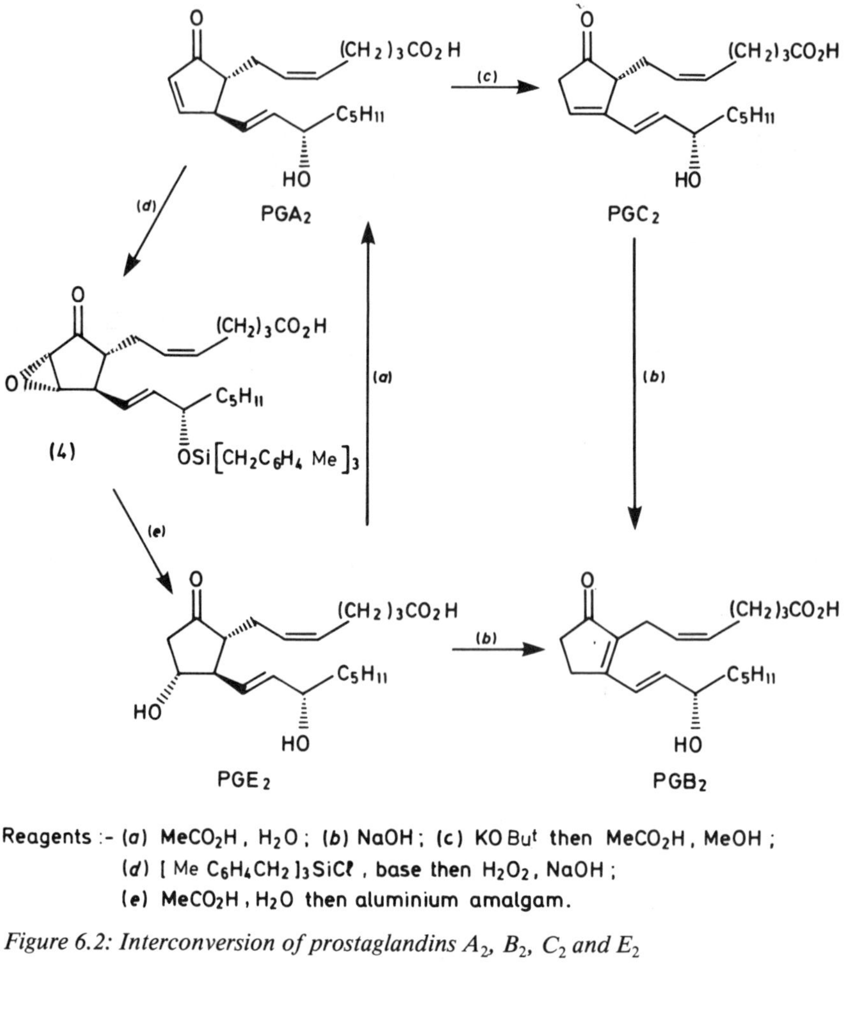

Reagents :- (*a*) $MeCO_2H$, H_2O; (*b*) NaOH; (*c*) $KOBu^t$ then $MeCO_2H$, MeOH;
(*d*) $[MeC_6H_4CH_2]_3SiCl$, base then H_2O_2, NaOH;
(*e*) $MeCO_2H$, H_2O then aluminium amalgam.

Figure 6.2: Interconversion of prostaglandins A_2, B_2, C_2 and E_2

Chemical interconversions of prostaglandins A, B, C and E

Acid-catalyzed dehydration of PGE_2 gave prostaglandin A_2 while base treatment of PGE_2 formed prostaglandin B_2 through the transient intermediacy of prostaglandin C_2 (PGC_2) (*see Figure 6.2*). PGC_2 may be obtained from PGA_2 by a deprotonation-reprotonation sequence under carefully controlled conditions[2].

The stereoselective conversion of A prostaglandins into E prostaglandins, as described in *Figure 6.2*, is important due to the ready availability of PGA_2-15-acetate from a Caribbean coral (*see* Chapter 1). The use of the tri-(*p*-xylyl)silyl group to protect the hydroxyl function at C-15 was crucial, since this group seemed to promote oxidation from the α-face of the five-membered ring to give (4). Removal of the silyl protecting group and reduction of the epoxide function using aluminium amalgam (the carbonyl function ensuring specific reduction at C-10) gave PGE_2 in 65 per cent yield from PGA_2.

Reduction of prostaglandins of the 2-series to prostaglandins of the 1-series

The 13,14-alkene linkage in prostaglandins is sterically more hindered than the 5,6-double bond. Thus, hydrogenation of $PGF_{2\alpha}$ or PGE_2 using Wilkinson's catalyst (tris-phenylphosphine rhodium (II) chloride) afforded $PGF_{1\alpha}$ or PGE_1 directly. Further protection of the 13,14-double bond is necessary if a palladium catalyst is used. Typically, PGE_2 was protected as the bis-dimethyl-isopropylsilyl ether, reduced with 5% palladium on charcoal under an atmosphere of hydrogen and deprotected to give PGE_1.

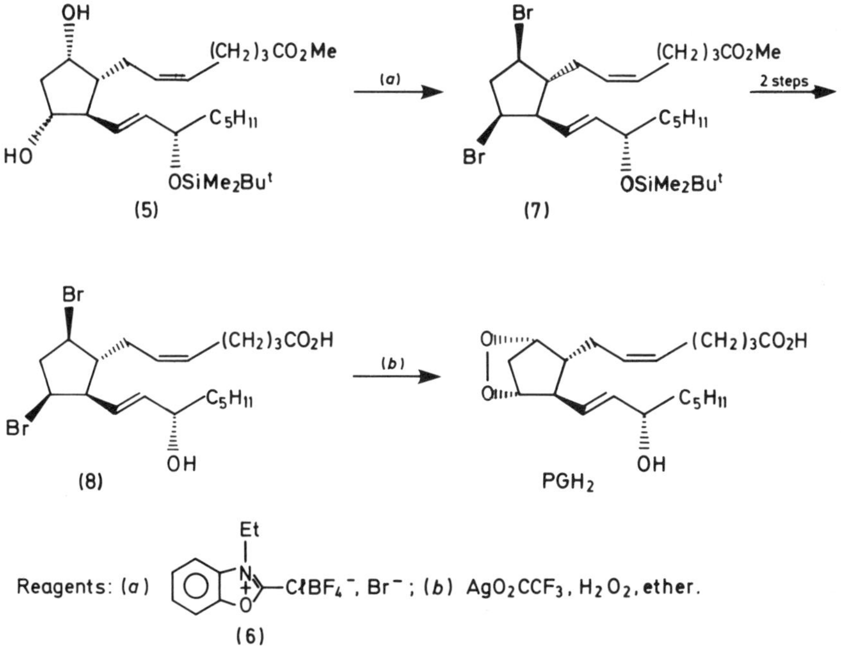

Reagents: (*a*) (6) $-C\ell BF_4^-$, Br^-; (*b*) AgO_2CCF_3, H_2O_2, ether.

Figure 6.3: Synthesis of prostaglandin H_2

Synthesis of prostaglandins G_2 and H_2

The endoperoxide prostaglandins H_2 (PGH_2) and G_2 (PGG_2) have attracted a great deal of attention because of their pivotal role in the biosynthesis of prostaglandins and because of their potent biological properties.

PGH_2 was prepared from 15-tert-butyldimethylsilyl-$PGF_{2\alpha}$ methyl ester (5) using the sequence described in *Figure 6.3*. 2-Chloro-3-ethylbenzoxazolium tetrafluoroborate (6) is the key reagent[3]. This compound activates alcohols towards halide displacement, such that the addition of bromide ion

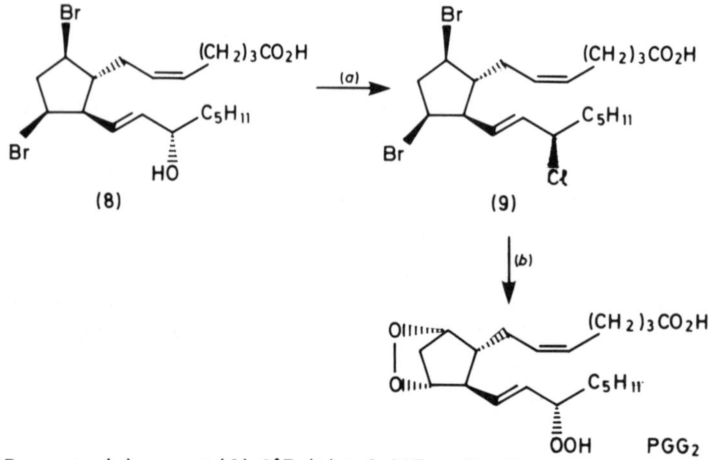

Reagents: (*a*) reagent (6), Cl^-; (*b*) AgO_2CCF_3, H_2O_2, ether.

Figure 6.4: Synthesis of prostaglandin G_2

to a solution containing (5) and (6) gave the 9β,11β-dibromo compound (7). Removal of the protecting groups and reaction of the dibromide (8) with hydrogen peroxide and silver trifluoroacetate in ether gave PGH_2 (*ca.* 7 per cent yield from $PGF_{2\alpha}$)[4].

PGG_2 can be prepared using a similar strategy (*see Figure 6.4*). Thus, the dibromide (8) was reacted with Mukaiyama's reagent (6) and chloride ion to give the trihalogeno compound (9): this compound was reacted with peroxide and a silver salt to give PGG_2 (*ca.* 6 per cent yield from $PGF_{2\alpha}$).

Synthesis of prostaglandin I_2

Prostaglandin I_2 (PGI_2) is formed from prostaglandins PGG_2 and PGH_2 by enzymes present in blood vessel walls. The ability of this prostaglandin to inhibit, and even reverse, the aggregation of blood platelets had caught the attention of many scientists. The complementary roles of thromboxane A_2 and prostaglandin I_2 in the cardiovascular system (*see* Chapters 3 and 7) and the possibility of using PGI_2 analogues in the prophylactic treatment of patients at risk from heart attack and stroke had led to the necessity for the chemist to find efficient routes to PGI_2[5].

Several synthetic routes to PGI_2 are available: all start from $PGF_{2\alpha}$ and all the routes are similar in strategy. The route described in *Figure 6.5* is typical. Treatment of $PGF_{2\alpha}$ with iodine in water containing sodium carbonate and potassium iodide gave the iodo ethers (10), (11), through the intermediacy of

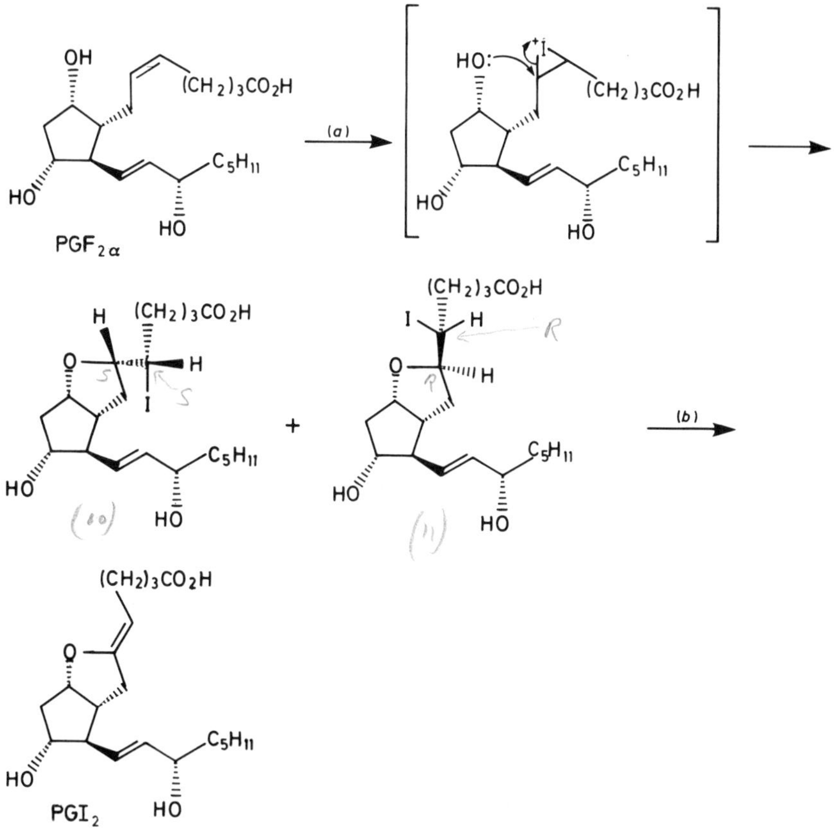

Reagents: (*a*) I_2, KI, Na_2CO_3, H_2O ; (*b*) DBN.

Figure 6.5: Synthesis of prostaglandin I_2

the iodonium ion and intramolecular etherification. *Trans*-elimination of the elements of hydrogen iodide was accomplished from both stereoisomers using the highly basic, non-nucleophilic amine, diazabicyclononene (DBN). The ester (12) was hydrolysed to the sodium salt of PGI_2 in standard fashion.

References

1. For further details see J.S. Bindra and R. Bindra, *Prostaglandin Synthesis,* Academic Press (New York), 1977, Chapter 18.
2. E.J. COREY and C.R. CYR, *Tetrahedron Lett.,* 1974, 1761.
3. T. MUKAIYAMA, S. SHODA and Y. WATANABE, *Chem. Lett.,* 1977, 383.
4. N.A. PORTER et al., *J. Am. chem. Soc.,* 1979, **101,** 4319; 1980, **102,** 1183.
5. K.C. NICOLAOU, G.P. GASIC and W.E. BARNETTE, *Angew. Chem. Int. Ed.,* 1978, **17,** 293.

CHAPTER 7

Synthesis of thromboxanes

Richard J.K. Taylor
School of Chemical Sciences, University of East Anglia, Norwich, Norfolk

Introduction[1]

In 1975, Bengt Samuelsson from the Karonlinska Institute in Stockholm showed[2] that incubation of the endoperoxides PGG_2 and PGH_2 with human blood platelets gave rise to the novel compound thromboxane A_2 (TXA_2) which was rapidly hydrolyzed to thromboxane B_2 (TXB_2) (*see* Chapter 2).

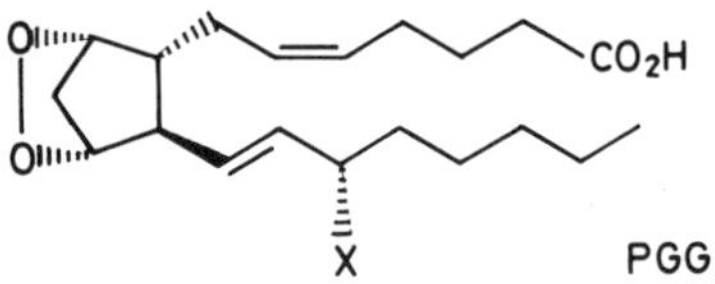

PGG_2 (X = OOH) ; PGH_2 (X = OH).

TXB_2 is stable and apparently possesses little biological activity. TXA_2, on the other hand, has a very short biological half life (approximately 32 seconds) which made characterization difficult. The bicyclic acetal structure was consistent with the labile nature of the compound and with the fact that hydrolysis gave the cyclic hemiacetal TXB_2. Additional proof was obtained by generating TXA_2 in the presence of various nucleophiles. The products obtained were in accord with nucleophilic attack occurring at the acetal carbon atom leading to opening of the strained oxetane ring.

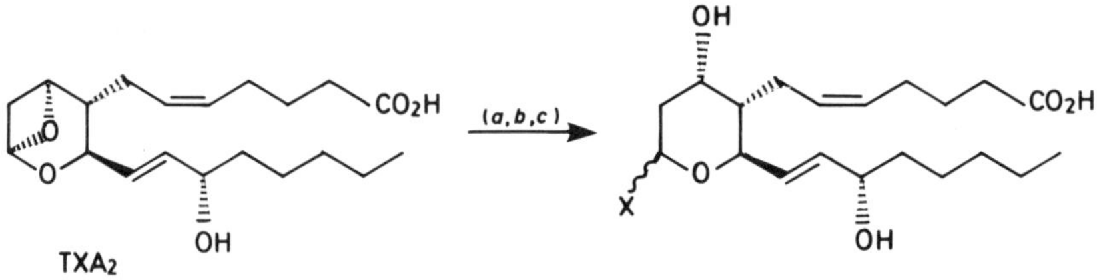

TXA_2 —(*a,b,c*)→

Reagents :- (*a*) MeOH ; (*b*) EtOH ; (*c*) NaN_3 ; with reagent (*a*) X = OMe ; with (*b*) X = OEt and with (*c*) X = N_3.

Although TXA_2 has not yet been isolated in pure form, it has generated an enormous amount of interest because of its striking cardiovascular properties. TXA_2 causes constriction of the blood vessels and is one of the most potent known aggregators of blood platelets (*see* Chapter 3).

In order to confirm the structures of the thromboxanes and obtain sufficient material to evaluate their wider biological roles, a number of synthetic approaches have been devised. To date, however, TXA_2 has not been prepared although several syntheses of TXB_2 have been published.

The syntheses fall into two major categories: first, those starting from prostaglandins or prostaglandin derivatives; and secondly, those starting from carbohydrates. One example from each of these categories is discussed in the following sections.

Synthesis of TXB_2 from prostaglandins and prostaglandin precursors

A group of chemists from the Upjohn Company published three syntheses of TXB_2 in 1976[3]. The synthesis devised by Schneider and Morge, which commenced with the $PGF_{2\alpha}$ derivative (1), is shown in *Figure 7.1.*

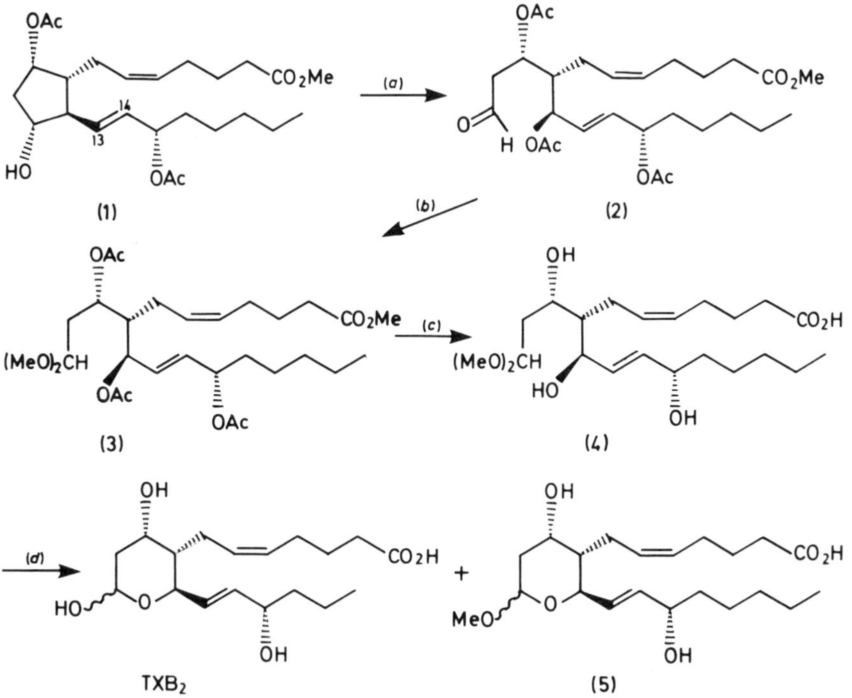

Reagents :- (*a*) $Pb(OAc)_4$, benzene, r.t.; (*b*) $(MeO)_3CH$, pyridine hydrochloride, MeOH; (*c*) HO^-/H_2O; (*d*) 85% phosphoric acid – H_2O–THF (1:10:12) (TXB_2, *ca.* 25% from 1).

Figure 7.1: Synthesis of TXB_2 by Schneider and Morge

The key step in this synthesis involves the opening of the cyclopentane ring in such a way that the product can be easily transformed into TXB_2. This was achieved by treating the methyl ester of 9,15-diacetoxy-$PGF_{2\alpha}$ (1) with lead tetraacetate (LTA). Lead tetraacetate is often used to cleave 1,2-diols: the accepted mechanism is outlined below.

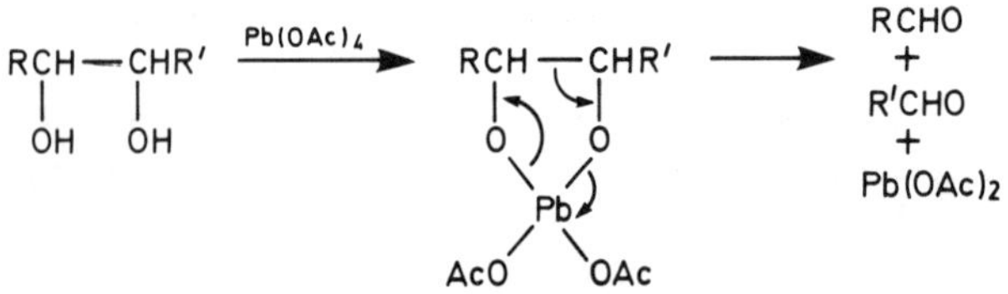

RCH—CHR' (OH, OH) $\xrightarrow{Pb(OAc)_4}$ RCH—CHR' (O, O; Pb; AcO, OAc) ⟶ RCHO + R'CHO + $Pb(OAc)_2$

The 13,14-double bond in (1) appears to facilitate the regiospecific fragmentation reaction leading to the acetoxyaldehyde (2). Protection of the aldehyde as an acetal, ester hydrolysis and finally acid-catalyzed acetal hydrolysis and intramolecular hemiacetal formation gave TXB_2 in 25 per cent yield from (1), together with a small amount of TXB_2 methyl acetal (5).

Synthesis from carbohydrates

The majority of natural products are optically active. In order to obtain the

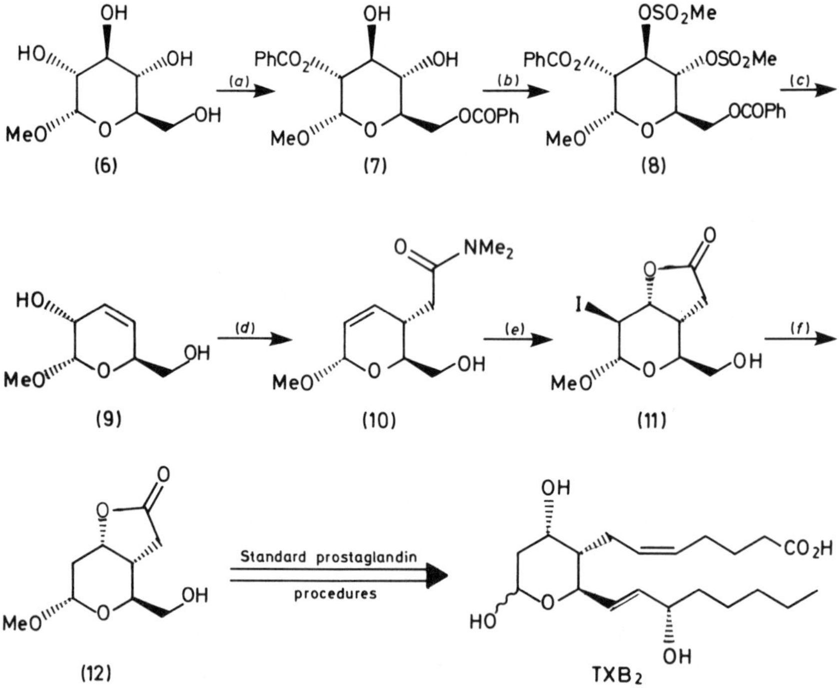

(6) —(a)→ (7) —(b)→ (8) —(c)→

(9) —(d)→ (10) —(e)→ (11) —(f)→

(12) —Standard prostaglandin procedures→ TXB_2

Reagents :- (a) PhCOCl, CH_2Cl_2, pyridine, − 30 °C (59%);
(b) $MeSO_2Cl$, pyridine, − 10 °C (93%);
(c) NaI, Zn(Cu), DMF, then MeOH, H_2O, Et_3N (35%);
(d) MeC $(OMe)_2NMe_2$, diglyme, 160 °C (75%);
(e) I_2, THF − H_2O, 0 °C (80%);
(f) Bu_3SnH (100%).

Figure 7.2: Chiral synthesis of TXB_2 intermediate (12)[4c]

natural enantiomer by conventional synthetic procedures, one of the racemic intermediates has to be resolved, and this can be wasteful in terms of both time and material. The problem can be avoided by employing an optically pure starting material; hexapyranose sugars, being inexpensive and readily available, are ideal precursors for TXB_2. Several groups[4] have used this approach for the synthesis of (+)-TXB_2; the preparation of the key optically active intermediate (12) from the methyl glycoside of *D*-glucose (6) by E.J. Corey's group is shown in *Figure 7.2*[4c].

Glycoside (6) was protected as the 2,6-dibenzoate (7) and then converted into the bis-methanesulphonate (8). This sequence illustrates the regioselectivity possible in the reactions of carbohydrates. Treatment of (8) with sodium iodide and a zinc-copper couple, followed by hydrolysis of the ester groups, gave the alkene (9). This elimination reaction presumably proceeded by the initial formation of a 1,2-diiodide:

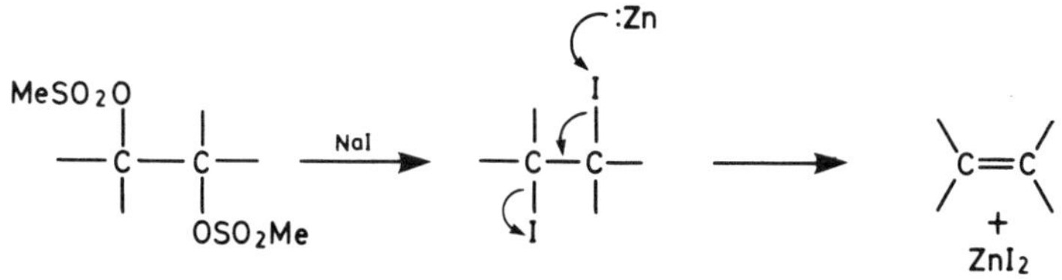

MeSO₂O–C–C–OSO₂Me —NaI→ I–C–C–I (:Zn) → C=C + ZnI_2

Reaction of (9) with *N,N*-dimethylacetamide dimethylacetal at 160°C gave the amide (10) by a Claisen rearrangement:

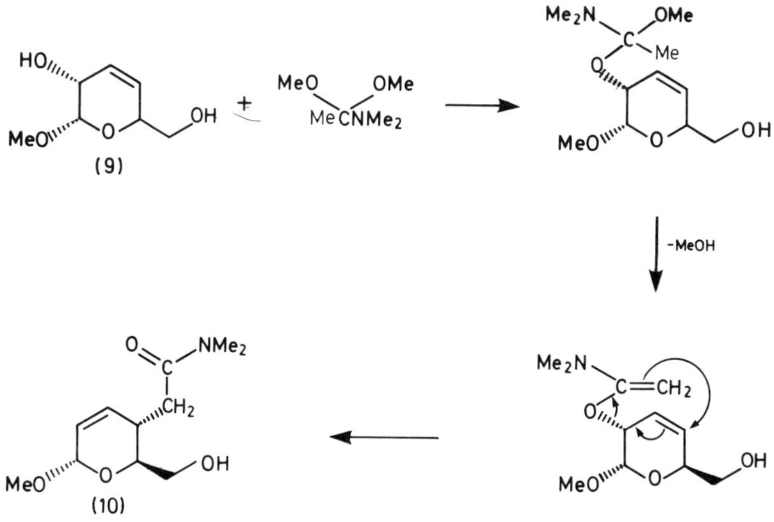

(9) + MeO, OMe, MeCNMe₂ → (−MeOH) → (10)

Amide (10) underwent cyclization when treated with aqueous iodide to give iodolactone (11).

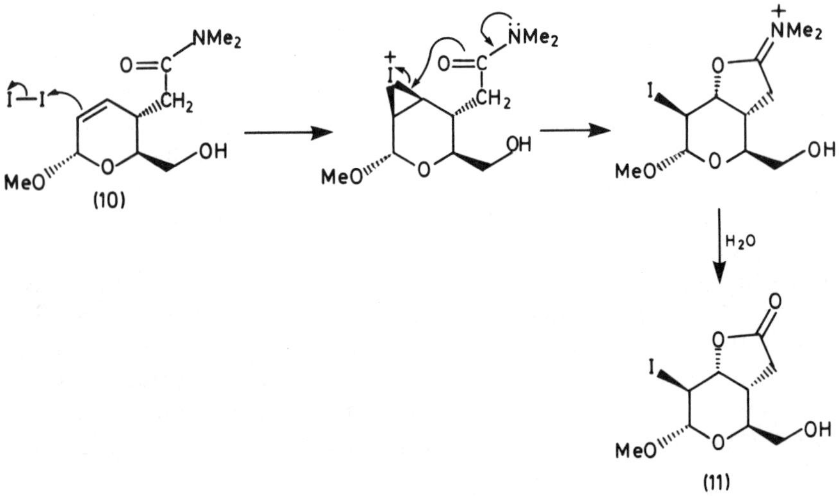

(10)

H_2O

(11)

Removal of the iodine using tri-n-butyl tin hydride gave the optically active intermediate (12) which could be converted into (+)-TXB_2 using standard prostaglandin reactions as listed in reference 3a.

References

1. For a more thorough review of the biological properties, biosynthesis and synthesis of the thromboxanes *see* K.C. Nicolaou, G.P. Gasic and W.E. Barnette, *Angew. Chem. Int. Ed.*, 1978, **17**, 293.
2. M. HAMBERG, J. SVENSSON and B. SAMUELSSON, *Proc. natn. Acad. Sci. U.S.A.*, 1975, **72**, 2994.
3. (a) N.A. NELSON, R.W. JACKSON, *Tetrahedron Lett.*, 1976, 3275; (b) R.C. Kelly, I. Schletter and S.J. Stein, *Tetrahedron Lett.*, 1976, 3279; (c) W.P. Schneider, R.A. Morge, *Tetrahedron Lett.*, 1976, 3283.
4. (a) S. HANESSIAN, P. LAVALLEE, *Can. J. Chem.*, 1977, **55**, 562; (b) H. Ohriu, S. Emoto, *Agric. biol. Chem.*, 1977, **41**, 1773; (c) E.J. Corey, M. Shabasaki, J. Knolle, *Tetrahedron Lett.*, 1977, 1625; (d) O. Hernandez, *Tetrahedron Lett.*, 1978, 219; (e) A.G. Kelly, J.S. Roberts, *J. Chem. Soc., Chem. Commun.*, 1980, 228.

CHAPTER 8

Synthesis and biological activity of prostaglandin analogues bearing modified side chains

Eric W. Collington
Chemical Research Department, Glaxo Group Research, Ware, Hertfordshire

Introduction

Much of the past decade's research seeking therapeutically useful prostanoids has been directed toward the preparation of structurally modified analogues which might possess greater tissue selectivity and be of longer duration in their action. The result has been the synthesis of a plethora of structures with biological activities differing somewhat from the natural materials. The majority of this work is described in the patent literature. Unfortunately, relatively few details of biological activity are available and structure-activity relationships in any series of compounds have rarely been revealed. Nonetheless, this chapter describes some of the highlights of studies on modified prostaglandins, centred on alterations of the alpha and omega chains of the natural materials.

Alkyl substituted analogues

The discovery that the initial step in the metabolism of the natural prostaglandins involves oxidation of the C-15 hydroxyl group to a ketone moiety by the enzyme 15-hydroxyprostaglandin dehydrogenase, led to the synthesis of 15-methyl substituted analogues, in which simple oxidation at C-15 was not possible. Although various syntheses of 15-methyl prostaglandins have been developed, (15*S*)-15-methyl-$PGF_{2\alpha}$ (1) is most conveniently prepared from $PGF_{2\alpha}$, as outlined in *Figure 8.1*. The conversion of 15-methyl-$PGF_{2\alpha}$ (1) into the 15-methyl-PGE_2 derivative (3) was made possible by the considerably different steric environment of the three hydroxyl groups of 15-methyl-$PGF_{2\alpha}$ methyl ester (2, R = H). Using a selective silylating reagent, trimethylsilyldiethylamine, the C-11 monosilyl derivative (2, $R = SiMe_3$) was obtained in nearly quantitative yield. Oxidation followed by removal of the protecting group gave (3) in 45 per cent overall yield.

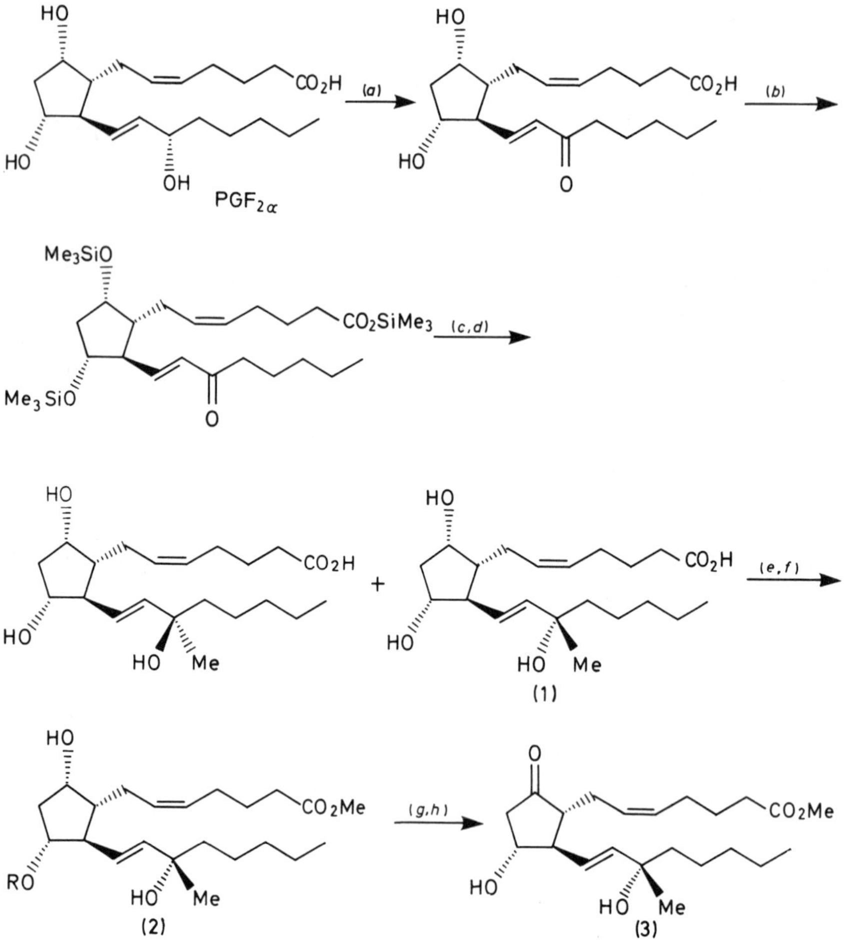

Reagents:- (*a*) DDQ; (*b*) Me_3SiCl, $(Me_3Si)_2NH$, THF; (*c*) MeMgBr, Et_2O; (*d*) aq.EtOH, 25 °C; (*e*) CH_2N_2; (*f*) Me_3SiNEt_2, acetone, −45 °C; (*g*) Collins reagent; (*h*) AcOH, MeOH.

Figure 8.1: Synthesis of 15-methyl $PGF_{2\alpha}$ and 15-methyl PGE_2

The presence of the 15-alkyl group does indeed render the compounds (1) and (3) inert to the action of 15-hydroxyprostaglandin dehydrogenase. Also, intrinsic prostaglandin activity is retained with both compounds in man, being significantly more potent in stimulating uterine contractility than their respective parent prostaglandins[1].

Alkyl substitution adjacent to the 15-hydroxyl group was also found to retard enzymatic oxidation. *Figure 8.2* summarizes the preparation of 16,16-dimethyl-PGE_2 (5) from the aldehyde (4). The PG analogue (5) is a potent antisecretory agent being 50 times more potent when given parenterally to dogs and much more potent in man than PGE_2. In addition it is orally active and has a prolonged duration of action[2].

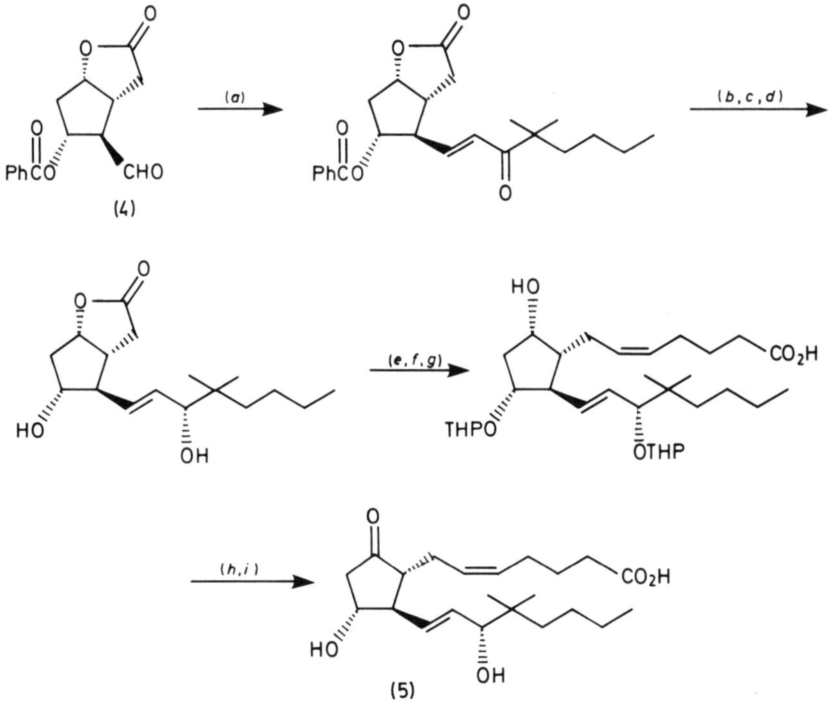

Reagents:- (*a*) $(MeO)_2\overset{+}{P}(O)\overset{-}{C}HCOC(Me_2)C_4H_9$; (*b*) $Zn(BH_4)_2$ (*c*) chromatographic separation; (*d*) K_2CO_3, MeOH; (*e*) DHP, PTSA; (*f*) Bu^i_2AlH; (*g*) $Ph_3PCH(CH_2)_3CO_2^-$; (*h*) Collins reagent; (*i*) H^+.

Figure 8.2: Synthesis of 16,16-dimethyl PGE$_2$

Dehydro analogues

Another way to diminish the ability of $PGF_{2\alpha}$ and PGE_2 to serve as 15-hydroxyprostaglandin dehydrogenase substrates is to convert the C-13,14-*trans*-double bond into a triple bond. *Figure 8.3* shows the synthesis of 13,14-dehydro-$PGF_{2\alpha}$ using the racemic bicyclic lactone (6) as starting material[3]. Reduction of lactone (6) with lithium aluminium hydride gave the diol, which was resolved into the desired natural material (7) *via* a bis-urethane formed by reaction with the isocyanate of (*R*)-α-phenylethylamine. It is noteworthy that regiospecific opening of the epoxide is achieved only by using a combination of the primary alcohol function in (7) and the t-butyl protected acetylenic alane (8), suggesting that the reaction probably proceeds *via* a cyclic-transition state favouring bond formation exclusively at C-12[4]. This change in the geometry and electronic properties at C-13 results in 13-dehydro-$PGF_{2\alpha}$ acting as an inhibitor of human placenta 15-hydroxyprostaglandin dehydrogenase. In addition, it is 5–10 times more potent than $PGF_{2\alpha}$ as an antifertility agent in the hamster.

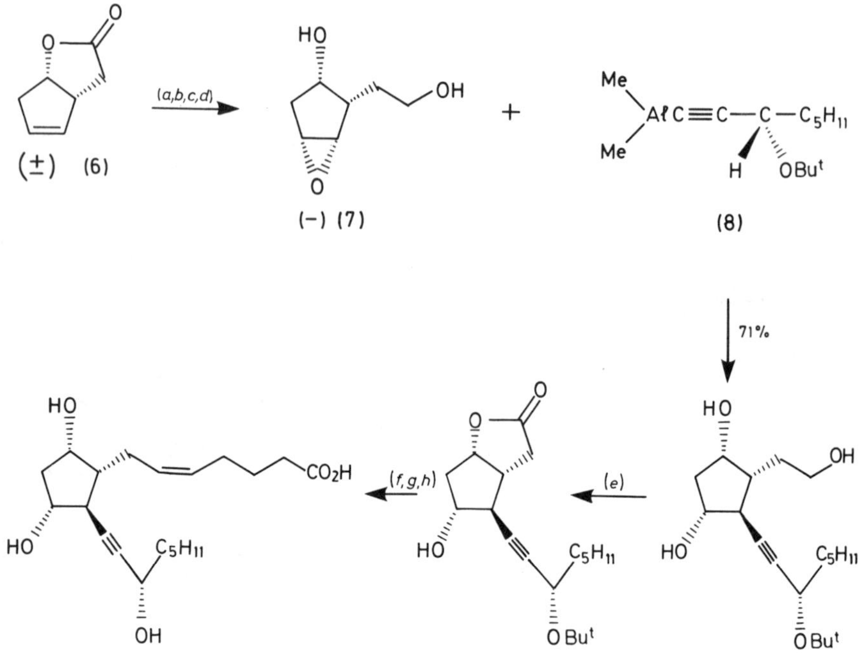

Reagents: (*a*) $LiAlH_4$; (*b*) (*R*)-α-PhCH(Me)NCO; (*c*) $LiAlH_4$; (*d*) MCPBA; (*e*) Pt, O_2, aq. acetone, $NaHCO_3$ (72%); (*f*) Bu^i_2AlH (87%); (*g*) $Ph_3PCH(CH_2)_3CO_2^-$; (*h*) TFA (93%).

Figure 8.3: Synthesis of 13,14-dehydro $PGF_{2\alpha}$

Aryloxy substituted analogues

During the past several years, a number of prostaglandin analogues have been synthesized which have incorporated an aryloxy group at some location in the prostaglandin structure. Two such examples are the 16-aryloxy-ω-tetranor prostaglandins (11) and (12). The regulation of luteal function as a means of controlling animal fertility is of considerable practical importance (*see* Chapter 3) and the search for compounds with greater luteolytic activity but less smooth muscle stimulant activity than $PGF_{2\alpha}$ has resulted in the development of the above compounds for veterinary use. When dosed subcutaneously to pregnant hamsters, ICI 80996 (cloprostenol) (11) and ICI 81008 (fluprostenol) (12) were, respectively, 200 and 100 times more potent than $PGF_{2\alpha}$ as luteolytic agents. *Figure 8.4* outlines the synthesis of both compounds from the aldehyde (10)[5]. The appropriate phosphonate reagent is readily prepared by reaction of an ester or an acid chloride with the anion (9).

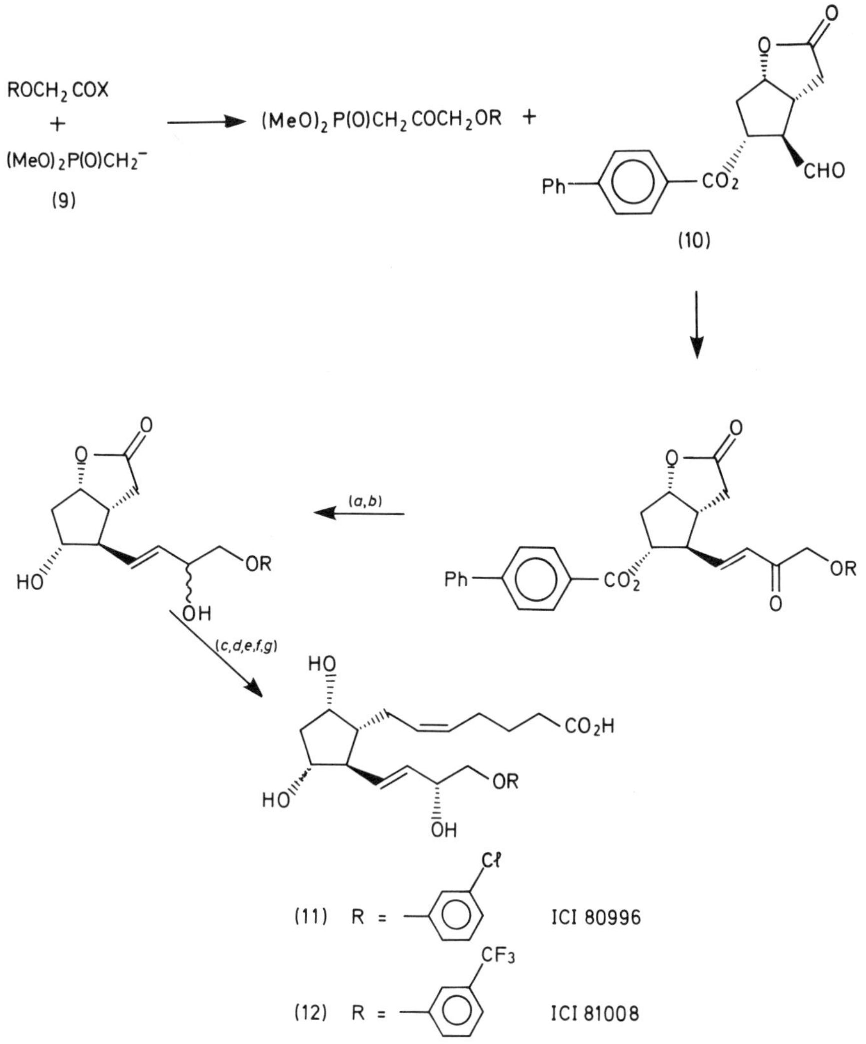

ROCH$_2$COX
+
(MeO)$_2$P(O)CH$_2^-$
(9)
→ (MeO)$_2$P(O)CH$_2$COCH$_2$OR +
Ph–C$_6$H$_4$–CO$_2$ ... CHO
(10)

(a,b)

OR
HO
OH
(c,d,e,f,g)

HO
CO$_2$H
HO
OR
OH

(11) R = 3-chlorophenyl ICI 80996

(12) R = 3-trifluoromethylphenyl ICI 81008

Reagents :- (a) Zn(BH$_4$)$_2$ (b) K$_2$CO$_3$, MeOH ; (c) DHP ; (d) Bu$^i_2$AlH ;
(e) Ph$_3$PCH(CH$_2$)$_3$CO$_2^-$; (f) H$^+$; (g) chromatography .

Figure 8.4: Synthesis of 16-aryloxy-ω-tetranor PGF$_{2\alpha}$

In an attempt to suppress both metabolic inactivation of the acid side-chain by β-oxidation and also metabolic alterations in the C-13 to C-15 region by a proximal steric effect, the inter-oxaphenylene PGE analogue (13) was prepared as shown in *Figure 8.5*[6]. The acid (13) is an extremely potent inhibitor of ADP-induced platelet aggregation in human platelet rich plasma, being about 30 times more potent than PGE$_1$.

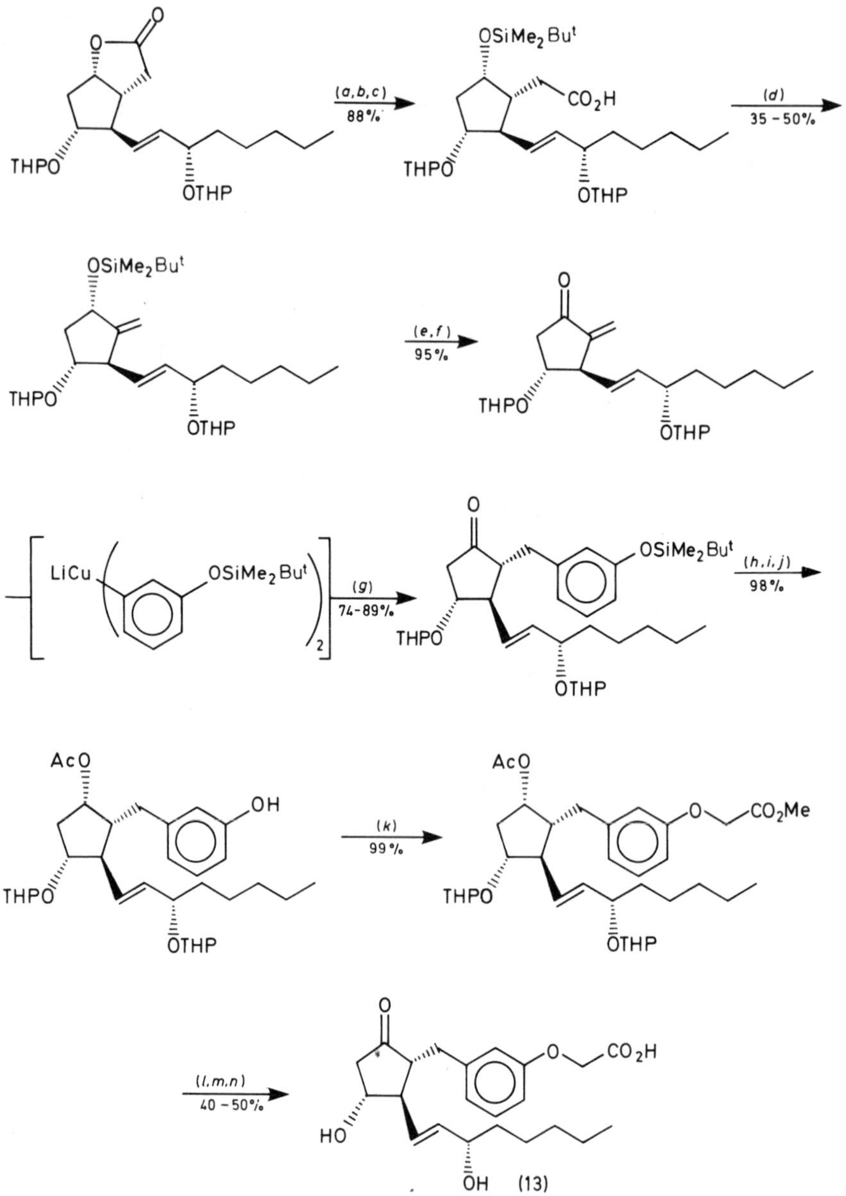

Reagents:- (*a*) NaOH, MeOH, H_2O, aq. $KHSO_4$; (*b*) Bu^t Me_2SiCl, imidazole, DMF; (*c*) K_2CO_3, MeOH, H_2O, aq. $KHSO_4$; (*d*) $Pb(OAc)_4$, $Cu(OAc)_2$, C_6H_6, pyridine, 80 °C; (*e*) Bu^n_4NF, THF; (*f*) H_2CrO_4, Me_2CO, −20 °C; (*g*) Et_2O, −78 °C; AcOH, Et_2O; (*h*) $NaBH_4$, MeOH, − 25 to −5 °C; (*i*) Ac_2O, pyridine, 4-DMAP; (*j*) Bu^n_4NF; (*k*) $BrCH_2CO_2Me$, NaH, $(MeOCH_2)_2$, 0 °C; (*l*) KOH, MeOH, H_2O, 40 °C (*m*) H_2CrO_4, Me_2CO, − 30 to −15 °C; (*n*) H_3PO_4, aq. THF, 35 °C.

Figure 8.5: Synthesis of PGE_2 with modified C_3–C_6 region

Heteroatom substituted analogues

A wide variety of other prostaglandin congeners incorporating a heteroatom in one of the side chains have been prepared. Although relatively little information is available concerning their quantitative biological activity, some of the synthetic approaches employed possess noteworthy features. For instance, in the synthesis of the 3-thia-PGE$_1$ analogue (17) (*see Figure 8.6*), the key intermediate (16) is obtained by rearrangement of the alkyl 2-furancarbinol (14)[7]. The increasing feature of this process is the effective isomerization of the 3-hydroxy isomer (15) to the desired 4-hydroxycyclopentenone (16) presumably by acid-catalyzed addition-elimination reactions.

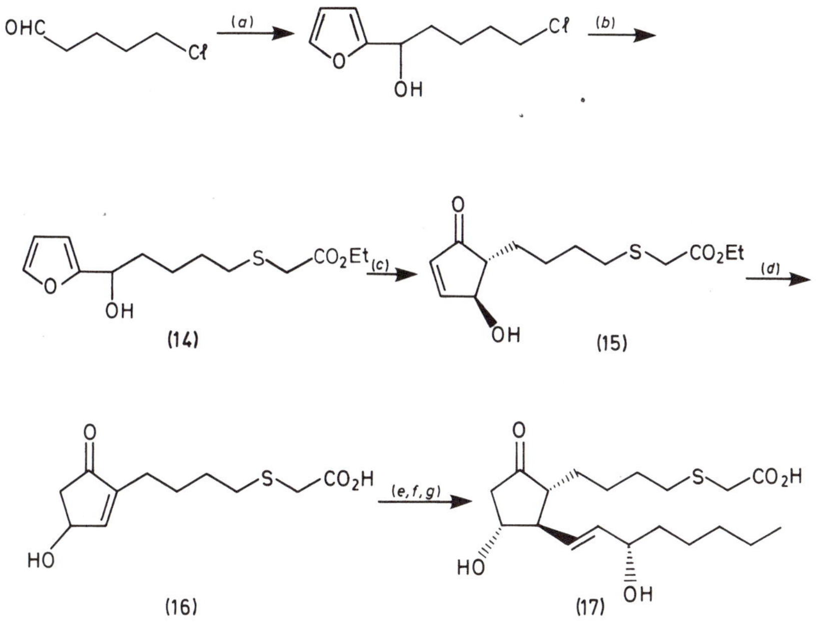

Reagents: (*a*) 2-furyl-Li, THF, −78 to 0 °C; (*b*) $NaSCH_2CO_2Et$, EtOH; (*c*) 2N HCO_2H, aq. dioxane, heat; (*d*) 0·5M H_2SO_4, aq. dioxan, heat; (*e*) DHP, PTSA; (*f*) Li[$C_3H_7C{\equiv}CCu$ $CH_2{=}CHCH(OSiEt_3)C_5H_{11}$]; (*g*) H^+.

Figure 8.6: Synthesis of 3-thia PGE$_1$

Figure 8.7 outlines a synthesis of the 13-aza-PGA$_2$ analogue (22)[8]. Although S_N2' reactions can proceed with *syn-* or *anti-*stereochemistry, reaction of the aminoalcohol (19) with the bromolactone (18) leads

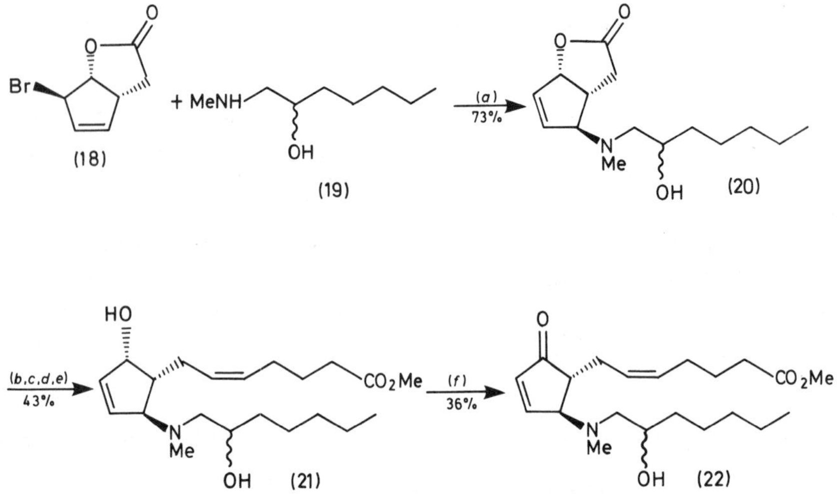

Reagents:- (*a*) MeOH, 25 °C; (*b*) Bu^i_2AlH, −78 °C; (*c*) $Ph_3PCH(CH_2)_3CO_2^-$, THF; conc. H_2SO_4, MeOH; (*d*) Ac_2O, pyridine; (*e*) K_2CO_3, MeOH; (*f*) H_2CrO_4, Me_2CO, 0 °C.

Figure 8.7: Synthesis of a 13-aza-PGA$_2$ analogue

exclusively to the *syn*-substituted product (20). Reduction of the lactone (20) with di-isobutylaluminium hydride and then a Wittig reaction followed by esterification and purification *via* the diacetate furnished the dihydroxy ester (21). Selective oxidation of the allylic alcohol using Jones reagent afforded the enone (22).

The Lepetit Company have recently described[9] a synthesis of 13-aza prostanoids commencing with the acid (23) (*see Figure 8.8*). Noteworthy in this synthesis is the condensation of the isocyanate (24) with a protected α-hydroxy acid to introduce directly the amide group into the lower chain. The conversion of the lactone (25) into the amido-prostaglandin analogue (26) was achieved by following classic organic reactions. The prostanoid (26) and some related analogues display potent abortifacient activity in pregnant hamsters.

C-1 Modified analogues

Prostaglandins in which the C-1 carboxy terminus has been changed to a biologically acceptable functionality or pro-drug equivalent have been prepared. One such example is the tissue selective *N*-acetyl-PGE$_2$-carboxamide (27) (*see Figure 8.9*), which has potent bronchodilatory activity following aerosol administration to asthmatic patients[10].

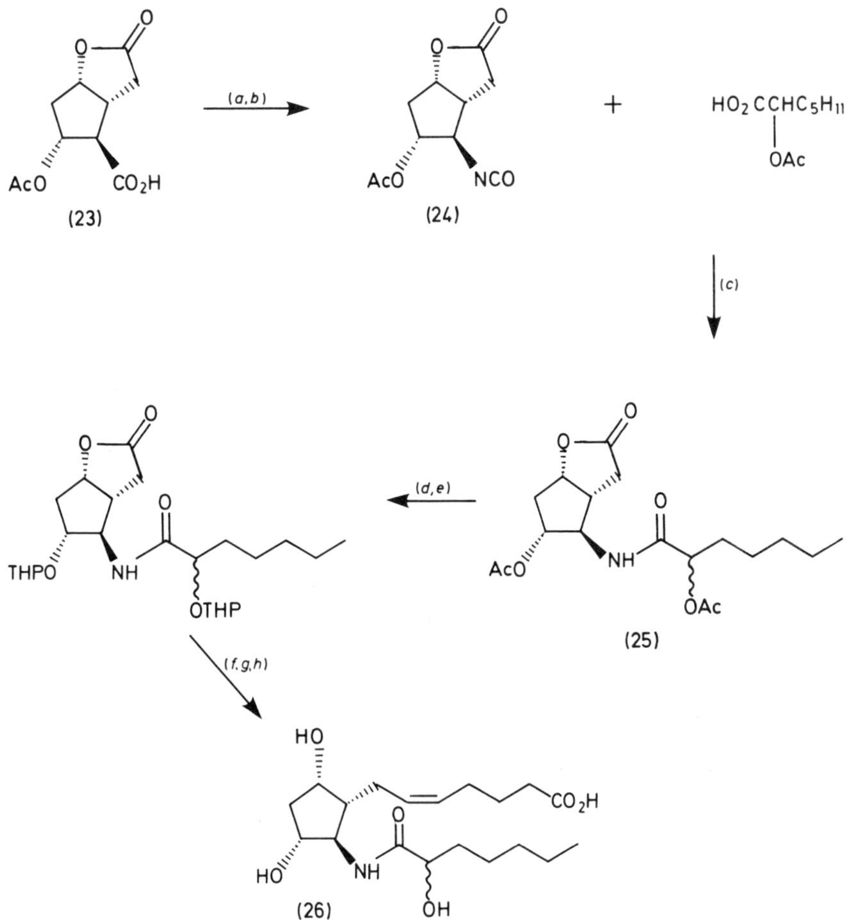

Reagents:- (*a*) Et_3N, $C\ell CO_2Et$, Me_2CO, NaN_3; (*b*) toluene, heat; (*c*) C_6H_6, pyridine, heat; (*d*) K_2CO_3, MeOH; (*e*) DHP, PTSA; (*f*) $NaA\ell H_2(OC_2H_4OMe)_2$, THF; (*g*) $Ph_3PCH(CH_2)_3CO_2^-$, DMSO; (*h*) $HC\ell$, Me_2CO.

Figure 8.8: Synthesis of a 13-aza-PGF$_{2\alpha}$ analogue

Synthesized in a similar manner, the PGE_2-tetrazole analogue (28) exhibited a pharmacological profile qualitatively and quantitatively similar to that of PGE_2[11].

Numerous *p*-substituted phenyl esters (30) of PGE_2 have been synthesized *via* the mixed anhydride (29) in an attempt to improve the solid state stability of the parent prostaglandin (*see Figure 8.10*). Evaluation showed that some esters provided increased stability in the solid state while still maintaining significant biological activity[12].

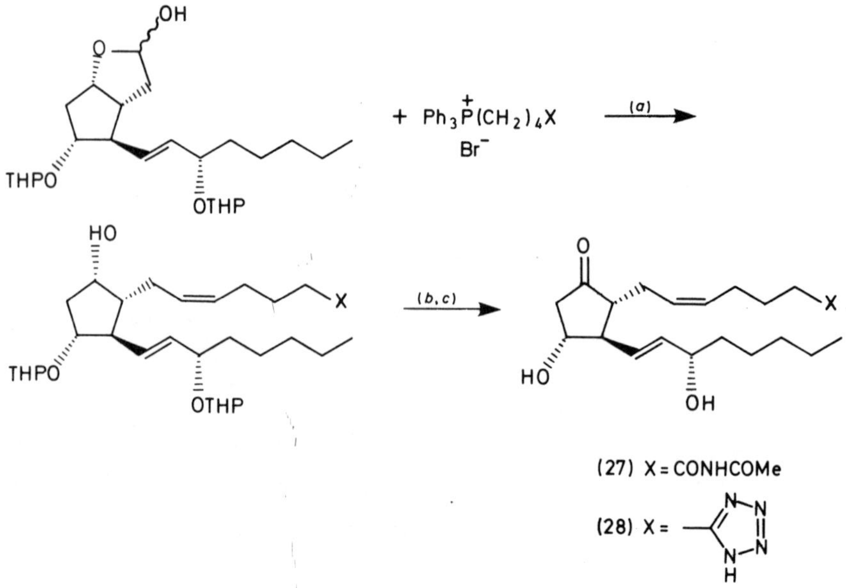

+ $Ph_3\overset{+}{P}(CH_2)_4X$ Br^- (a)

THPO OTHP OH O

HO THPO OTHP X (b, c)

O X HO OH

(27) X = CONHCOMe

(28) X = tetrazolyl (N–N=N–NH)

Reagents :- (a) $NaCH_2SOMe$, DMSO ; (b) H_2CrO_4, MeCO, 0 °C ; (c) AcOH, H_2O, 25 °C.

Figure 8.9: Synthesis of prostaglandin E_2 analogues incorporating an amide or a tetrazole moiety at C_1

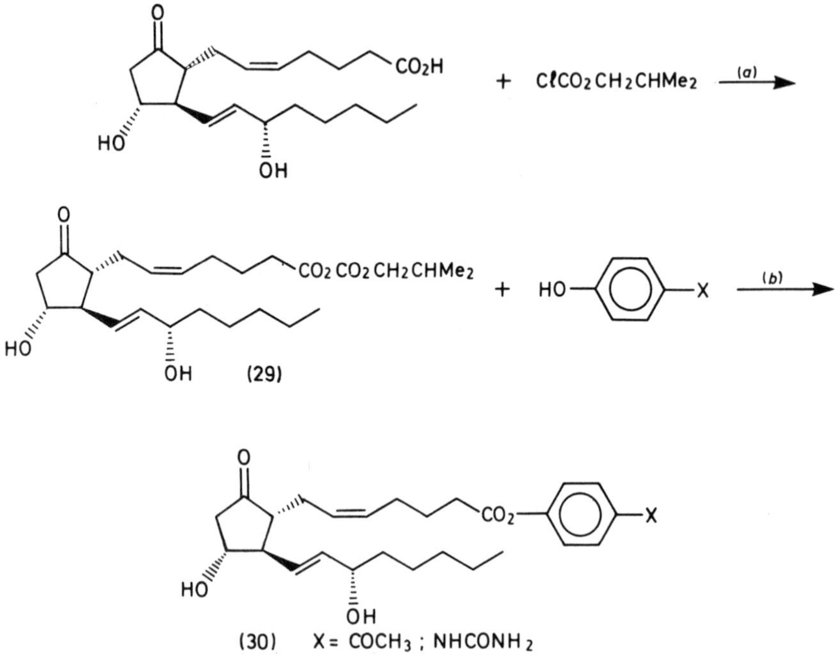

O CO_2H HO OH + $ClCO_2CH_2CHMe_2$ (a)

O $CO_2CO_2CH_2CHMe_2$ HO OH (29) + HO–C_6H_4–X (b)

O CO_2–C_6H_4–X HO OH

(30) X = $COCH_3$; $NHCONH_2$

Reagents :- (a) Et_3N, THF ; (b) pyridine, 25 °C.

Figure 8.10: Synthesis of some aryl-esters of PGE_2

Hybrid analogues

Although considerable promise of potential therapeutic activity has been shown by some of the many prostaglandin congeners synthesized that possess changes in either the alpha or omega side-chains, the search for high potency, tissue selectivity and metabolic stability has resulted in the synthesis of

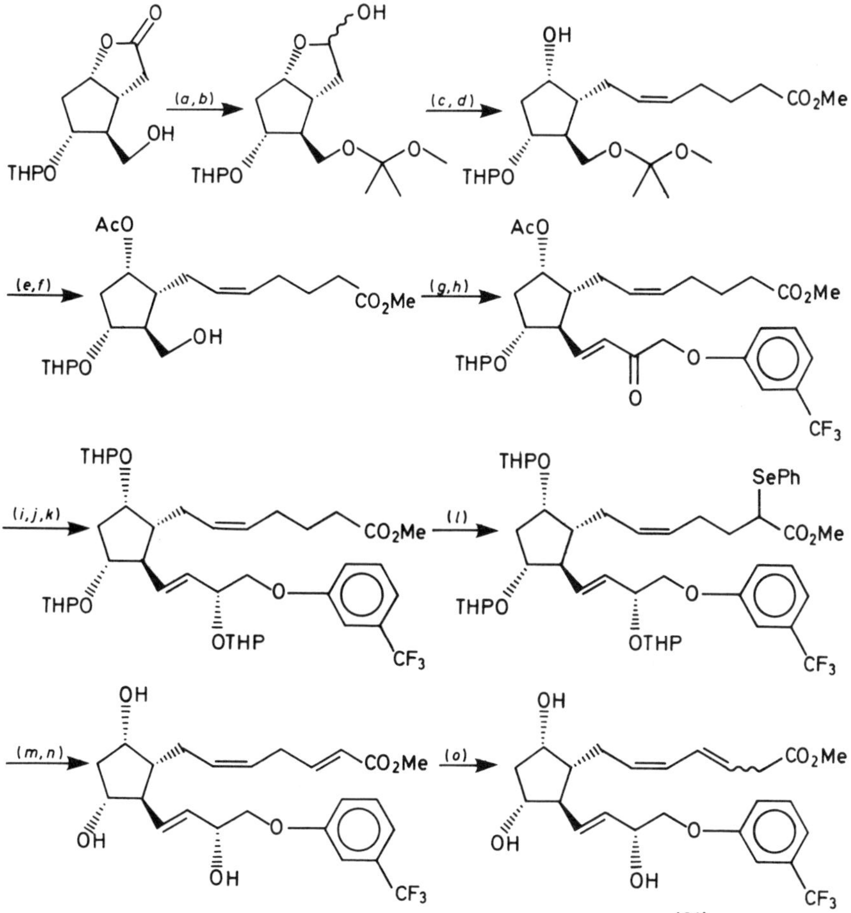

(31)

Reagents:- (*a*) 2-methoxypropene, PTSA, CH_2Cl_2; (*b*) $Bu^i{}_2AlH$; 100%;
(*c*) $NaCH_2SOMe$, $Ph_3\overset{+}{P}(CH_2)_4CO_2H.\ Br^-$; (*d*) K_2CO_3, MeI; 85%;
(*e*) Ac_2O, pyridine; (*f*) 0·5N HCl, THF, 0 °C; 89%; (*g*) SO_3-pyridine, DMSO; 90%; (*h*) NaH, $(MeO)_2P(O)CH_2COCH_2OC_6H_4CF_3$, THF, 43%;
(*i*) $NaBH_4$, MeOH, chromatography; 36%;
(*j*) K_2CO_3, MeOH; (*k*) DHP, PTSA; 91%; (*l*) LDA, PhSeSePh, THF; 64%;
(*m*) 30% H_2O_2, EtOAc, MeOH; 85%; (*n*) 65% aq. AcOH, THF; 71%;
(*o*) K_2CO_3, MeOH, 0 °C; 95%.

Figure 8.11: Synthesis of a 3,5-diene-16-aryloxy $PGF_{2\alpha}$ analogue

numerous analogues containing simultaneous structural changes in both chains.

In pursuit of potent antinidatory prostanoids, an examination of the effect of additional double bonds introduced into the alpha chain in relationship to other changes in the omega chain resulted in the synthesis of the 3,5-diene-16-aryloxy-$PGF_{2\alpha}$ analogue (31)[13] (*see Figure 8.11*). This analogue (which is a 2:1 mixture of *trans*-Δ^3-*cis*-Δ^5: *cis*-Δ^3-*cis*-Δ^5 compounds) exhibited an antinidatory effect in the rat 1200 times more potent than $PGF_{2\alpha}$. Interestingly, this 2:1 mixture (31) was found to be more potent than the individual components, presumably resulting from their synergistic effect.

The synthesis, although lengthy, illustrates an example of useful complementary methods for protection/deprotection of hydroxyl groups, so often a fundamental requirement in prostaglandin synthesis.

References

1. (a) M. BYGDEMAN, F. BEGUIN, M. TOPPOZADA, W. WIQVIST AND S. BERGSTROM, *Lancet,* 1972, **1,** 1336, (b) S.M.M. Karim and S.D. Sharma, *J. Obstet. Gynaec. Br. Commonw.,* 1972, **79,** 737.
2. A. ROBERT, B. NYLANDER and S. ANDERSSON, Life Sci., 1974, **14,** 533.
3. J. FRIED, M.S. LEE, B. GAEDE, J.C. SIH, Y. YOSHIKAWA and J.A. McCRACKEN, *Adv. Prostaglandin Thromboxane Res.,* 1976, **1,** 183.
4. J. FRIED, J.C. SIH, C.H. LIN and P. DALVEN, *J. Am. chem. Soc.,* 1972, **94,** 4343.
5. D. BINDER, J. BOWLER, E.D. BROWN, N.S. CROSSLEY, J. HUTTON, M. SENIOR, L. SLATER, P. WILKINSON and N.C.A. WRIGHT, *Prostaglandins,* 1974, **6,** 87.
6. D.R. MORTON and J.L. THOMPSON, *J. org. Chem.,* 1978, **43,** 2102.
7. C.V. GRUDZINSKAS, J.S. SKOTNICKI, S.L. CHEN, M.B. FLOYD, JR., W.A. HALLETT, R.E. SCHAUB, G.J. SIUTA, A. WISSNER, M.J. WEISS and F. DESSY, *Drugs Affecting the Respiratory System,* A.C.S. Symposium Series 118, 1980, 301.
8. E.W. COLLINGTON, H. FINCH, R.F. NEWTON and C.J. WALLIS, GB 2028805A.
9. Gruppo Lepetit Spa, DT 2705797.
10. S.L. SPECTOR and R.E. BALL, JR., *Ann. Allergy,* 1977, **38,** 302.
11. N.A. NELSON, R.W. JACKSON and A.T. AU, *Prostaglandins,* 1975, **10,** 303.
12. W. MOROZOWICH, T. O. OESTERLING, W. L. MILLER, C. F. LAWSON, J. R. WEEKS, R. G. STEHLE and S. L. DOUGLAS, *J. pharm. Sci.,* 1979, **68,** 833.
13. M. HAYASHI, Y. ARAI, H. WAKATSUKA, M. KAWAMURA, Y. KONISHI, T. TSUDA and K. MATSUMOTO, *J. med. Chem.,* 1980, **23,** 525.

CHAPTER 9

Synthesis and biological activity of prostaglandin analogues with modified ring systems

Roger P. Dickinson
Pfizer Central Research, Pfizer Ltd., Sandwich, Kent

Introduction

A vast amount of effort has been expended on the synthesis of modified prostaglandins with the aim of overcoming the problems shown by the natural compounds, namely, lack of selectivity and oral activity, poor duration of action, and chemical instability. Much of the effort has centred on modifications to the ring system and it is the purpose of this chapter to highlight some of the main trends in this area.

Unfortunately it is not always possible to evaluate the effect of structural modification on biological activity since, for many analogues, no biological results have been reported. Even where results are quoted, the use of different test systems and procedures often makes comparison difficult. Nevertheless, sufficient information is available to conclude that appropriate modification of the ring system can sometimes lead to compounds with sufficient activity and selectivity of action to be considered for clinical evaluation. However, where compounds have been tested in man the results so far have proved disappointing.

Incorporation of additional ring substituents

Prostaglandins of the E series readily dehydrate to PGAs which, in turn, are transformed chemically and, in some species at least, enzymically to PGCs. The latter are further isomerized to the biologically inactive PGBs (*see* Chapter 6 and *Figure 9.1*).

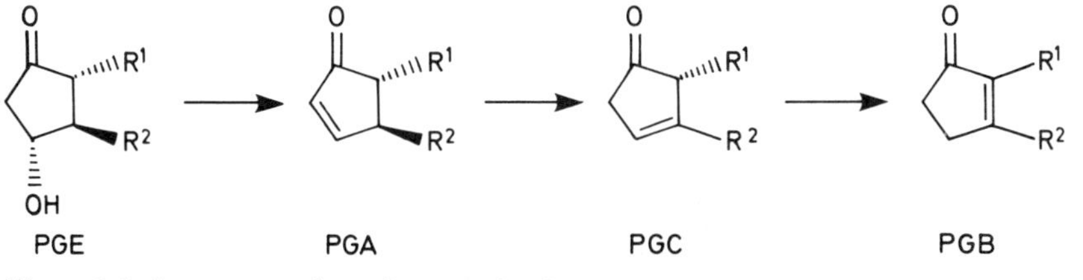

PGE PGA PGC PGB

Figure 9.1: Interconversion of prostaglandins A, B, C, and E

Introduction of additional substituents has been used as a means of blocking each step in this sequence with the aim of achieving a more prolonged action. Thus, 10,10-dimethyl-PGE_1(1), which cannot dehydrate to a PGA derivative, has been prepared. The only activity reported for it is very weak stimulation of isolated rat uterus[1].

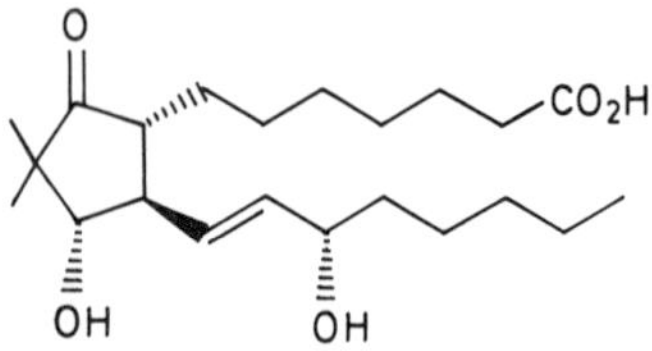

(1) 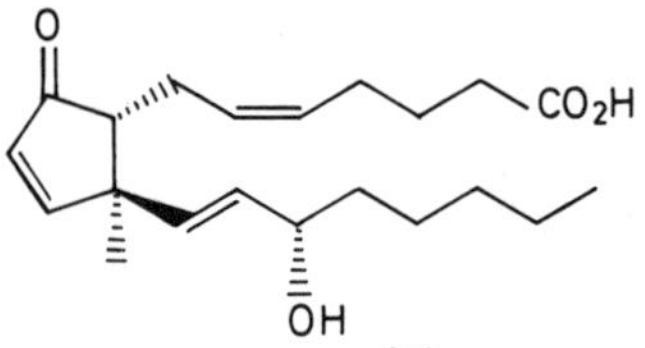 (2)

Introduction of a methyl group at C-12 of PGA_2 has been used as a means of blocking the isomerization to PGC_2. The synthesis of 12-methyl-PGA_2 (2) was carried out by Corey and co-workers[2]. 12-Methyl-PGA_2 was found to have no effect on blood pressure in dogs, nor did it inhibit gastric acid secretion in rats.

Corey has also reported the synthesis of 8-methyl-PGC_2 (5), in which the final isomerization step in the sequence of *Figure 9.1* is blocked[3]. The route summarized in *Figure 9.2* was used.

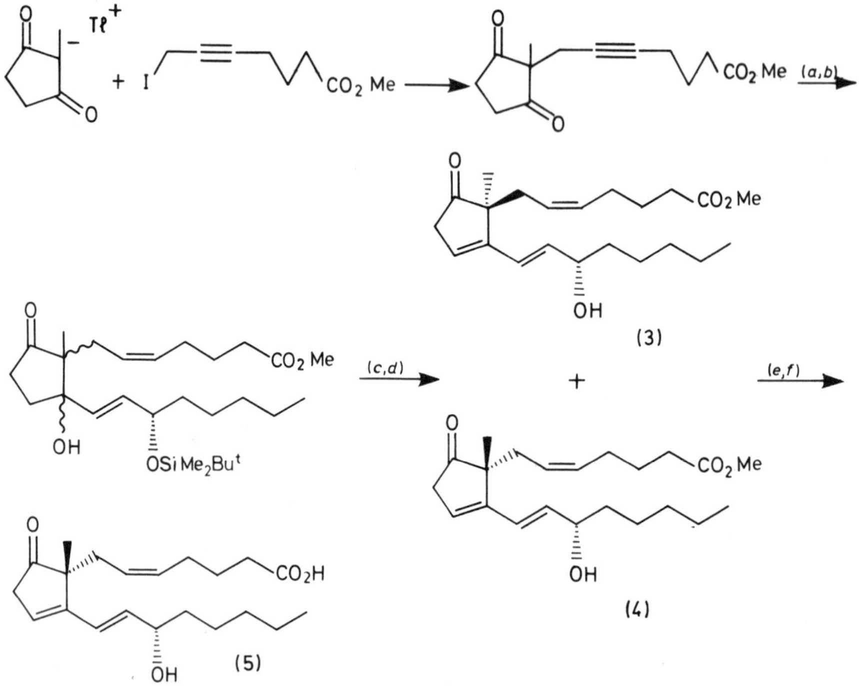

(3) (4) (5)

PT 9·2 Reagents :- (*a*) H_2, Lindlar catalyst; (*b*) LiCH=CHCH ($OSiMe_2Bu^t$)C_5H_{11};
(*c*) $SOCl_2$, C_5H_5N, CH_2Cl_2; (*d*) AcOH, THF, H_2O;
(*e*) chromatography; (*f*) porcine pancreatic lipase.

Figure 9.2: Synthesis of 8-methyl PGC_2

8-Methyl-PGC_2 (5) has 0.03 times the activity of PGE_2 on isolated smooth muscle. The intermediate esters (3) and (4) had about half the activity of PGE_2 or PGA_2 in inhibiting gastric acid secretion in rats.

The major points of metabolic attack in prostaglandins are in the side chains, and introduction of additional substituents into the ring would not normally be expected to affect this.

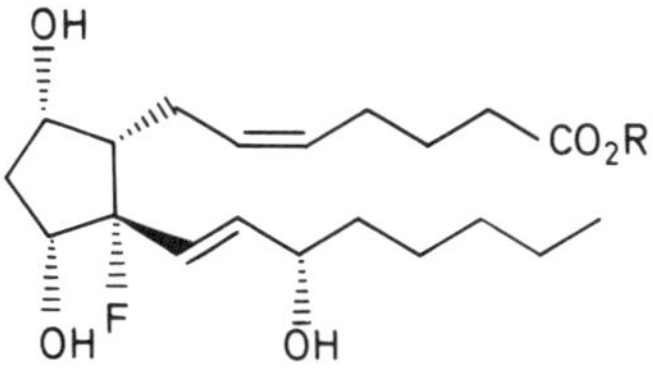

(6) R = Me
(7) R = H

However, the ester (6) was 12.5 times more potent than $PGF_{2\alpha}$ as a luteolytic agent in hamsters; this was attributed, at least in part, to the fact that the compound is not a substrate for the 15-hydroxyprostaglandin dehydrogenase enzyme[4]. In addition it was found that smooth muscle stimulant activity was markedly diminished and (6) had only 0.28 and 0.001 times the *in vitro* activity of $PGF_{2\alpha}$ on hamster uterine strips and gerbil colon, respectively[4]. The corresponding acid (7) had 25 times the luteolytic activity of $PGF_{2\alpha}$, while showing a similar selectivity profile to the ester[5].

12-Methyl-$PGF_{2\alpha}$ (8) was also prepared, but no activity has been reported for it.

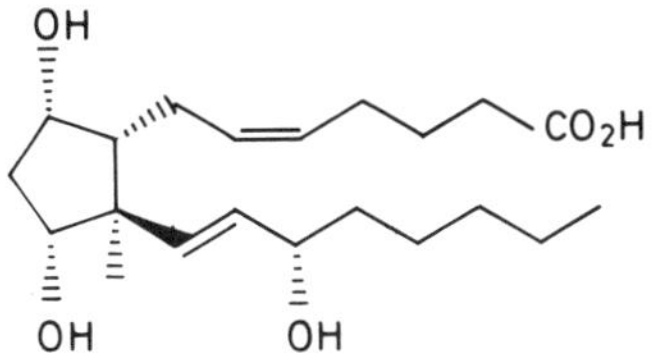

(8)

Deoxyprostaglandins

Analogues of PGEs lacking the hydroxyl group at C-11 are no longer degradable by the sequence shown in *Figure 9.1*. This fact, coupled with their relative structural simplicity, has made 11-deoxyprostaglandins attractive synthetic targets and many syntheses have been reported[6,7]. The majority of syntheses involve conjugate addition to a 2-cyclopentenone substituted in the α-position by the complete acidic side chain or a suitable precursor. A typical approach is that of Bagli and Bogri in which the cyclopentenone ester (9) is converted into the aldehyde (10), thereby allowing introduction of the omega side chain by a conventional Wittig route. Alternatively, the complete omega side chain may be introduced in protected form as in the method of Sih and co-workers (*see Figure 9.3*).

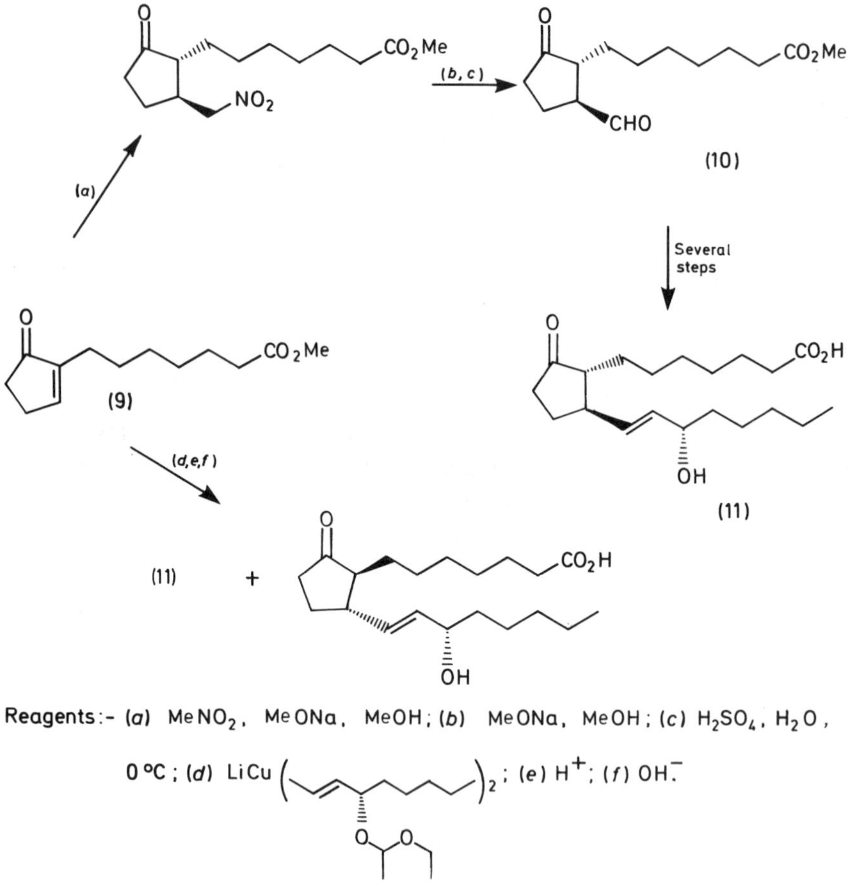

CO2Me
(b, c)
NO2
CO2Me
CHO
(10)
(a)
Several steps
CO2Me
(9)
CO2H
OH
(11)
(d,e,f)
(11)
+
CO2H
OH
Reagents:- (a) MeNO2, MeONa, MeOH; (b) MeONa, MeOH; (c) H2SO4, H2O,
0 °C; (d) LiCu ( )2; (e) H+; (f) OH−

Figure 9.3: Synthesis of 11-deoxyprostaglandin E_1 (11)

The cyclopentenone precursors have been prepared by several routes. A high yielding synthesis of (9) by Novak and Szantay is outlined in *Figure 9.4*.

11-Deoxy-PGE$_2$ methyl ester (12) has been prepared in 47 per cent overall yield by Patterson and Fried, using a short convergent route involving conjugate addition of a cuprate derivative of the protected omega side chain to 2-cyclopentenone, followed by trapping of the resultant enolate by silylation. The acidic side chain was introduced by regeneration of the lithium enolate followed by alkylation (*see Figure 9.5*). Attempts to alkylate the initially-formed enolate directly were unsuccessful.

An alternative approach to 11-deoxyprostaglandins is exemplified by the synthesis of Corey and Ravindranathan outlined in *Figure 9.6*. The key step in this route is the Tl^{III} promoted rearrangement of the cyclohexene lactone (13) to the cyclopentane aldehyde (14), which was then elaborated by conventional means to 11-deoxy-PGE$_2$ (15) and 11-deoxy-PGF$_{2\alpha}$ (16).

11-Deoxyprostaglandins are also available from reduction of PGA$_2$ (17) and ester derivatives. Thus, 11-deoxy-PGE$_1$ (11) has been prepared by

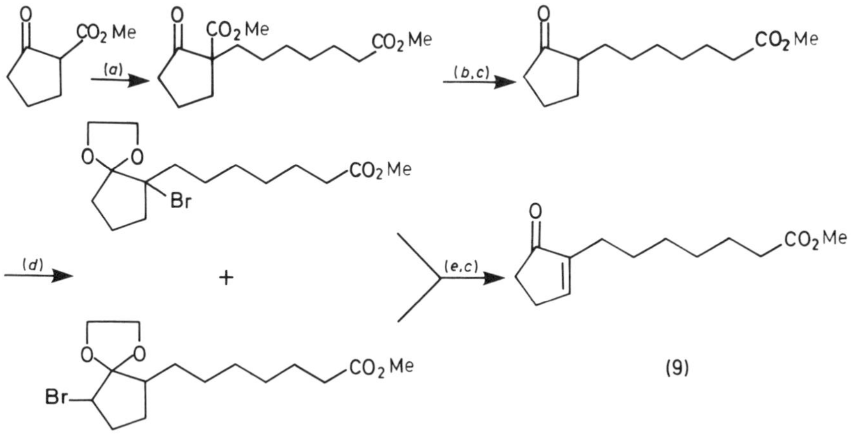

Reagents:- (*a*) $Br(CH_2)_6CO_2Me$, K_2CO_3, acetone; (*b*) H_2SO_4, H_2O, reflux; (*c*) MeOH, C_6H_6, H^+; (*d*) Br_2, $HO(CH_2)_2OH$; (*e*) NaOH, MeOH, reflux.

Figure 9.4: Preparation of 1-methoxycarbonylhexylcyclopent-2-enone

hydrogenation of PGA_2 in the presence of Wilkinson catalyst, whereas sodium borohydride reduction gave a mixture of 11-deoxy-$PGF_{2\alpha}$ (16) and 11-deoxy-$PGF_{2\beta}$ (18) (*see Figure 9.7*).

The *in vivo* bronchodilator effects of 11-deoxyprostaglandins have been studied in detail and an interesting structure-activity pattern has been found[8]. 11-Deoxy-PGE_1 has similar broncodilator activity to PGE_1 after aerosol administration to guinea-pigs, but 11-deoxy-PGE_2 has only 0.001 times the activity of PGE_2. 11-Deoxy-$PGF_{2\alpha}$(16) is at least 10 times more active than $PGF_{2\alpha}$ as a bronchoconstrictor.

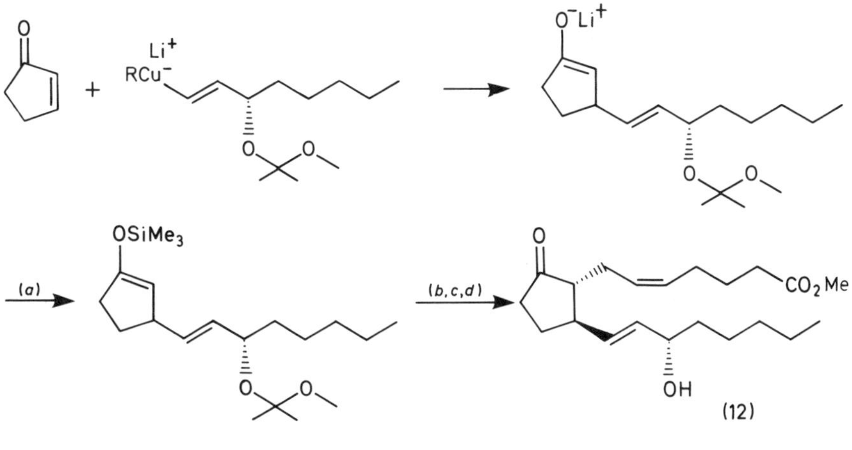

Reagents:- (*a*) $ClSiMe_3$; (*b*) Li/NH_3; (*c*) $BrCH_2CH{=}CH(CH_2)_3CO_2Me$; (*d*) AcOH, MeOH, H_2O.

Figure 9.5: Short convergent route to 11-deoxy PGE_2 methyl ester

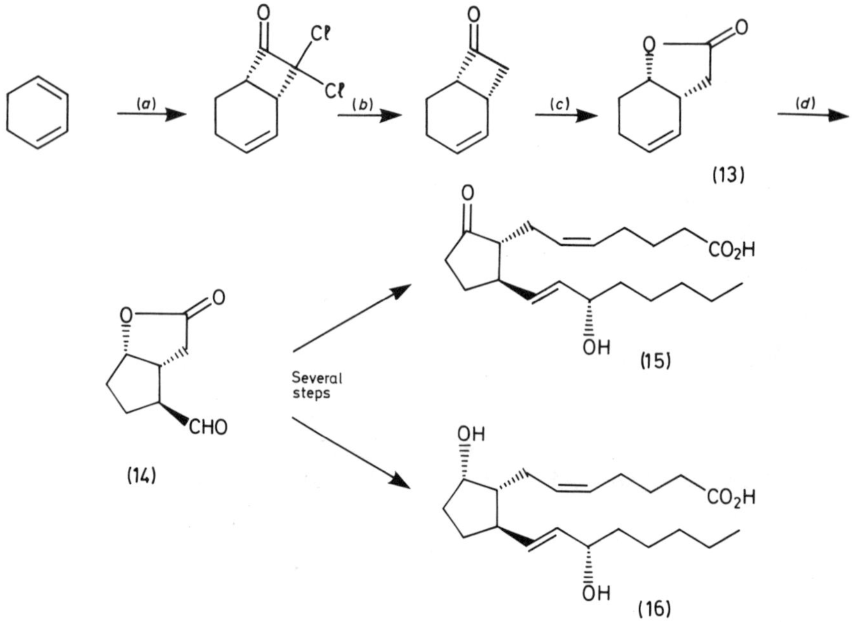

(13)

(15)

Several steps

(14)

(16)

Reagents:- (*a*) dichloroketen; (*b*) Zn, AcOH; (*c*) H_2O_2, MeOH, H_2O, pH 10; (*d*) $Tl(NO_3)_3$, H_2O, $HClO_3$, $NaClO_3$.

Figure 9.6: Synthesis of 11-deoxy-PGs by Corey et al.

Several 11-deoxyprostaglandins have been examined for their effect on gastric acid secretion[9]. Ketone (19), a mixture of C-15 epimers of 11-deoxy-PGE_1, had one tenth the antisecretory activity of PGE_1 in rats. The corresponding PGF analogue (20) was about eight times less active than (19). Modification of the omega side chain to hinder metabolism by the

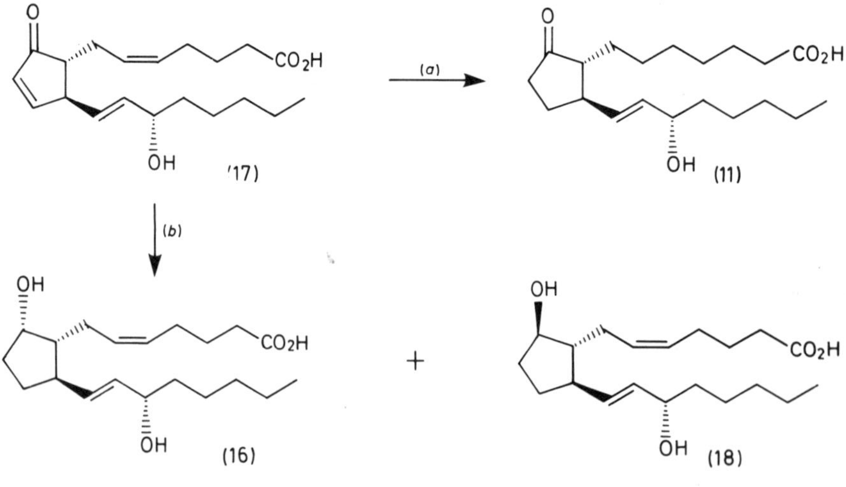

(17)

(11)

(16)

(18)

Reagents:- (*a*) H_2, Wilkinson catalyst, EtOH, C_6H_6; (*b*) $NaBH_4$.

Figure 9.7: Preparation of 11-deoxy PGs from PGA_2

15-hydroxyprostaglandin dehydrogenase enzyme led to compounds with greater potency and duration of action after oral administration, a typical example being the ketone (21). Hybrid analogues incorporating modifications in both side chains are also known. For example, the Pfizer compound (22) inhibits histamine-, pentagastrin- and food-stimulated gastric acid secretion in dogs after both oral and intravenous administration and inhibits gastric ulceration in rats when given intravenously[10].

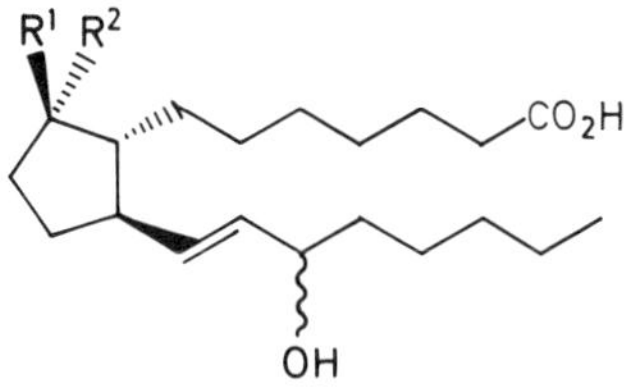

(19) $R^1, R^2 = O$
(20) $R^1 = H, R^2 = OH$

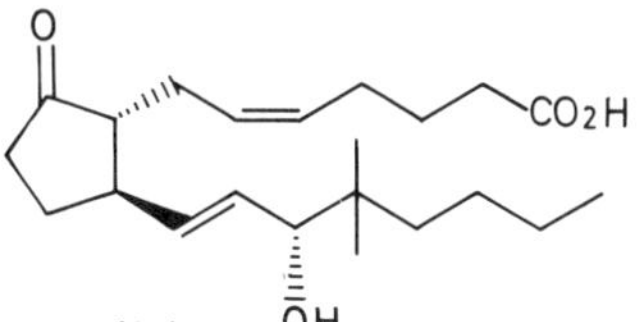

(21)

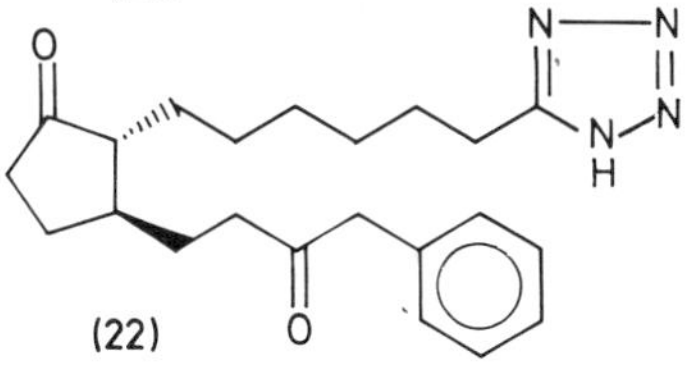

(22)

9-Deoxyprostaglandins have been less studied but several analogues are known. Workers at Ciba-Geigy have prepared 9-deoxy-PGE_1 (24) starting from the readily available cyclopentenone ester derivative (23)[11].

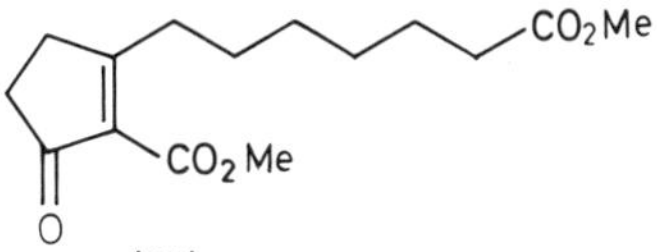

(23)

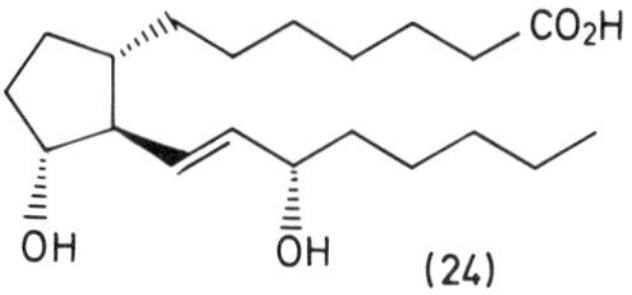

(24)

9-Deoxy-PGE_1 (24) was claimed to have prostaglandin-like activity, but the test systems used have not been reported.

Deoxyprostaglandins with additional substituents

The availability of PGA_2 esters from the Caribbean coral *Plexaura homomalla* has made PGA_2 and its simple derivatives attractive starting materials for the synthesis of novel prostanoids. This is particularly true for 11-substituted-11-deoxyprostaglandins, which can be readily prepared by addition reactions to the cyclopentenone system (*see Figure 9.8*).

Thus, treatment of PGA_2 methyl ester (25; $R = CH_3$) with lithium dimethylcuprate, followed by hydrolysis, gives 11-deoxy-11α-methyl-PGE_2 (26) in 70 per cent yield[12]. Treatment of (25; $R = CH_3$) with thiols in the presence of triethylamine gives mixtures of 11α- and 11β-alkylthio-11-deoxy-PGE_2 derivatives (27), which are separable by chromatography[12, 13]. Other substituents which have been introduced by Michael-type addition reactions include CH_2NO_2, CN, $CH{=}CH_2$ and $SCOCH_3$.

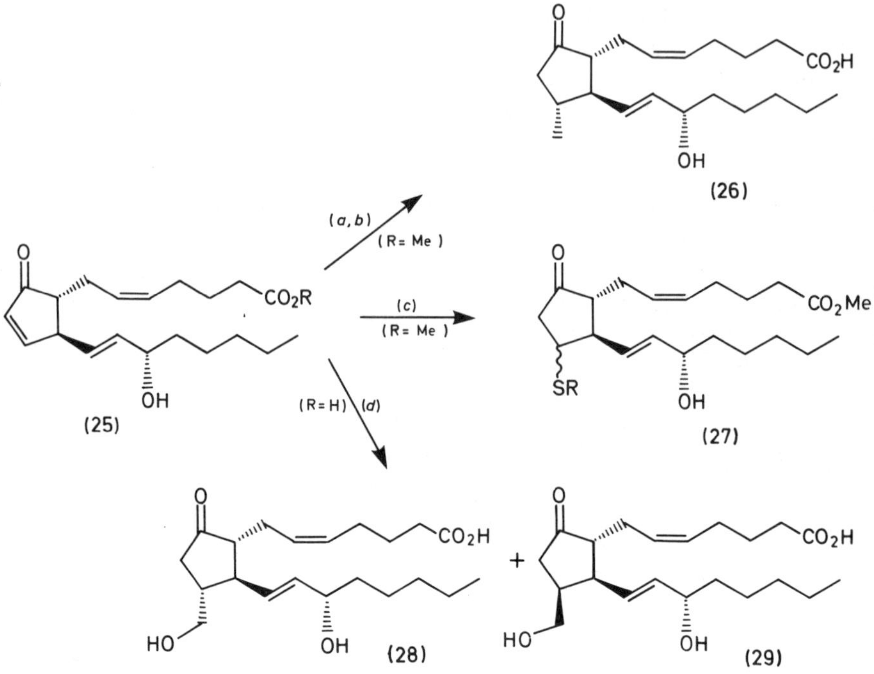

Reagents :- (*a*) Me_2CuLi ; (*b*) hydrolysis ; (*c*) RSH, Et_3N ; (*d*) MeOH, Ph_2CO, $h\nu$.

Figure 9.8: Some routes to 11-substituted 11-deoxy PGS

Benzophenone-sensitized photo-addition of methanol to PGA_2 (25; R = H) gives an 80 per cent yield of a 4:1 mixture of 11α- (28) and 11β-hydroxymethyl-11-deoxy-PGE_2 (29), which are separable by chromatography[14]. Total syntheses of (28) and the corresponding PGE_1 analogue have also been reported.

11-Substituted-11-deoxy-PGF derivatives have been prepared by reduction of the PGE analogues with $NaBH_4$, but mixtures of the 9α- and 9β-hydroxy compounds result. Greater selectivity for the 9α-products is achieved by using the more bulky reducing agent lithium perhydro-9β-boraphenalyl hydride (*see* Chapter 6 and *Figure 9.9*)[12].

11-Deoxy-11-halogeno- and 9-deoxy-9-halogeno-prostaglandins have been

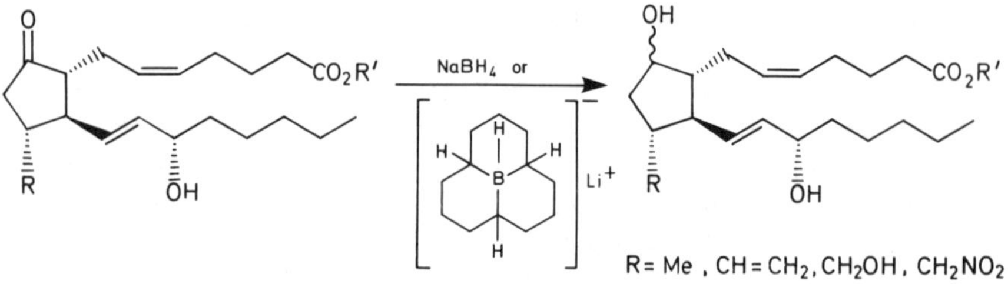

R = Me, $CH=CH_2$, CH_2OH, CH_2NO_2

Figure 9.9: Reduction of 11-deoxy PGEs to 11-deoxy PGFs

prepared by workers at Syntex[15]. Fluoro substituted compounds were prepared by replacement of a hydroxyl group in a suitably protected PGF_2 derivative with fluorine using diethyl (2-chloro-1,1,2-trifluoroethyl)amine. Replacement of hydroxyl by chlorine was accomplished using triphenylphosphine in carbon tetrachloride. In each case, introduction of the halogen occurs with inversion of configuration. The approach is illustrated by the preparation of the 9β-chloro- and 9β-fluoro-analogues (30) and (31) (*see Figure 9.10*).

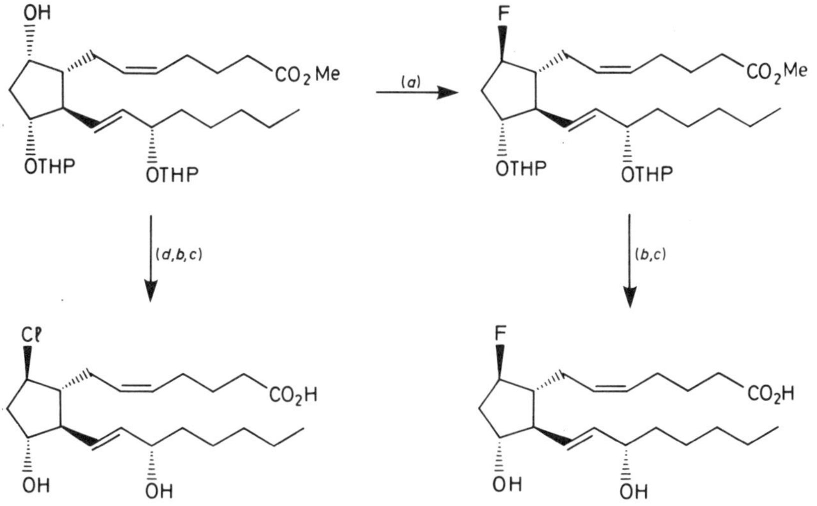

(30) (31)

Reagents:- (*a*) Et_2NCF_2CHClF; (*b*) AcOH, H_2O; (*c*) K_2CO_3, H_2O, MeOH; (*d*) CCl_4, Ph_3P, DMF, 35 °C.

Figure 9.10: Preparation of 9β-halogeno-9-deoxy-$PGF_{2\alpha}$

11-Deoxy-11α-hydroxymethyl-PGE_1 (32) was found to be equiactive with $PGF_{2\alpha}$ in causing contraction of rat uterus, but was markedly less active as a diarrhoeal agent. The corresponding PGE_2 analogue (28) showed comparable activity[16].

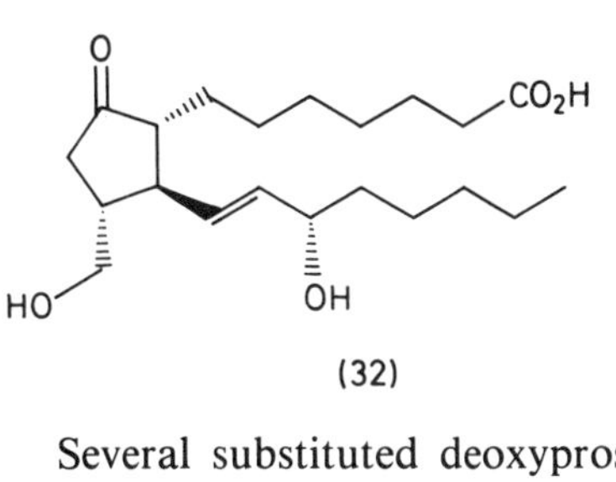

(32) 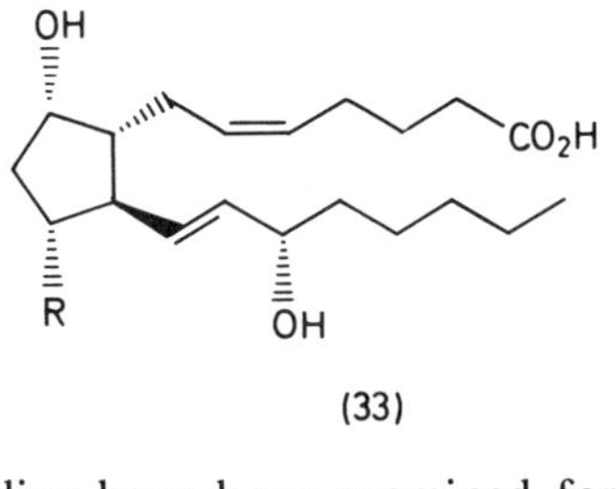 (33)

Several substituted deoxyprostaglandins have been examined for their effect on bronchial smooth muscle[8]. 11-Deoxy-11α-methyl-PGE_2 (26) had only 0.01 times the bronchodilatory activity of PGE_2 after aerosol administration to guinea-pigs. However, greater activity is shown by the thioether derivative (27; R = α-SCH_2CH_2OH) which is reported to have 0.15 times the activity of PGE_2 in guinea-pigs[13]. It is also active in dogs after aerosol administration and has no cardiovascular side effects. Removal of the hydroxyl group (27; R = SCH_2CH_3) or extension of the side chain (27; R = $SCH_2CH_2CH_2OH$) led to a marked reduction in activity.

The 11-substituted 11-deoxy-$PGF_{2\alpha}$ analogues (33; R = CH_3) and (33; R = CN) are at least as potent as $PGF_{2\alpha}$ in causing bronchoconstriction in guinea-pigs after aerosol administration[8]. In marked contrast, the fluoro analogue (33; R = F) was found to have bronchodilatory activity one tenth that of PGE_2 after intravenous administration. The 11β-fluoro isomer had negligible activity, but the 11β-chloro analogue was half as active as (33; R = F)[15]. It is not known if the bronchodilatory action of the halo analogues is due to an intrinsic different in activity or is a result of the different route of administration.

The 9-deoxy-9β-fluoro compound (31) had four times the bronchodilatory activity of PGE_2 after intravenous administration, and 2.5 times the activity after aerosol administration. The 9β-chloro analogue (30) had half the activity of PGE_2 when given as an aerosol while the 9α-fluoro analogue had only 0.05 times the activity. Because of its potency, (31) was chosen for clinical investigation but unfortunately it caused upper airway irritation in man[15].

Additional fused rings

Several analogues are known in which an additional ring has been fused onto the cyclopentane ring[17]. The 10,11-methylene compound (34) has been prepared by the route outlined in *Figure 9.11*.

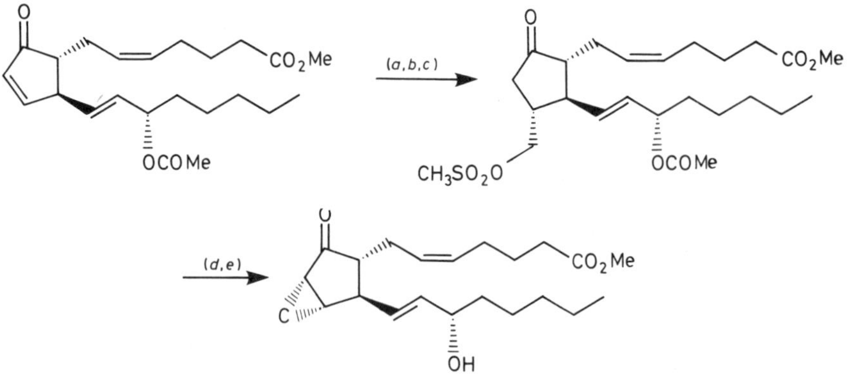

O

CO_2Me

OCOMe

(a, b, c)

O

CO_2Me

CH_3SO_2O

OCOMe

(d, e)

O

CO_2Me

C

OH

(34)

Reagent: (*a*) MeOH, Ph_2CO, $h\nu$; (*b*) chromatography to remove 11β-epimer; (*c*) $MeSO_2Cl$, Et_3N, CH_2Cl_2; (*d*) 1,5-diazabicyclo[5.4.0]undec-5-ene; (*e*) K_2CO_3, MeOH.

Figure 9.11: Synthesis of 10,11-methylene-11-deoxy PGE_2 methyl ester

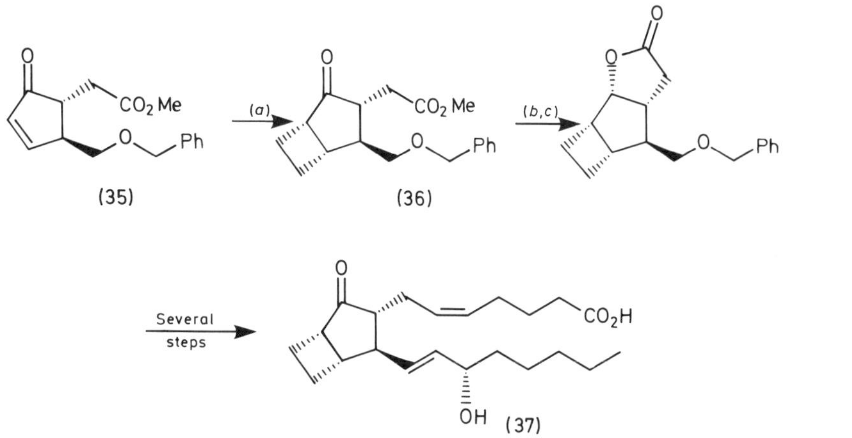

(35) (36) (37)

Reagents: (*a*) ethylene, $h\nu$, CH_2Cl_2, -70 °C; (*b*) $NaBH_4$; (*c*) H^+.

Figure 9.12: Synthesis of 10,11-ethylene-11-deoxy PGE_2

Crabbé and co-workers have synthesized the 10,11-ethylene derivative (37). The key step in this synthesis was the [2+2] photo-cycloaddition of ethylene to the enone (35) to give (36) which was then converted into the product (37) using standard prostaglandin methodology (*see Figure 9.12*).

A 10,11-trimethylene analogue (40) has been prepared using a synthesis in which the key step was generation of the fused cyclopentenone system (39) by treatment of the alkyne-cobalt complex (38) with cyclopentene. The omega side chain was then introduced by conjugate addition to give (40) (*see Figure 9.13*)[18].

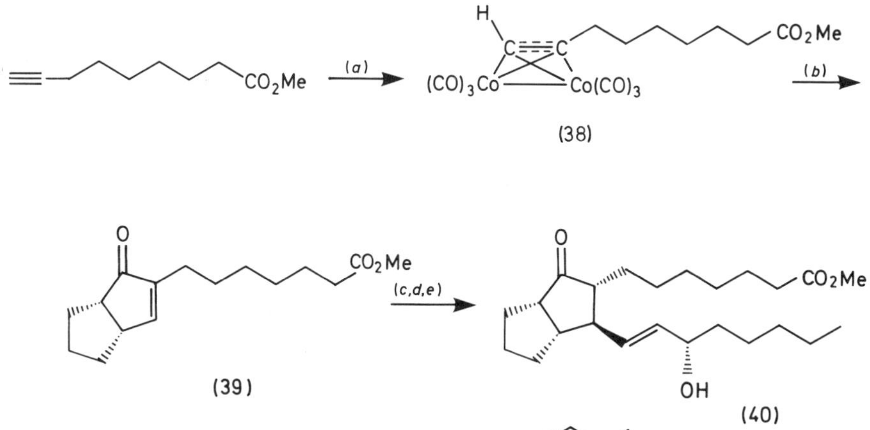

(38) (39) (40)

Reagents: (*a*) $Co_2(CO)_8$; (*b*) cyclopentene; (*c*) LiCu(C≡C–C_3H_7)(CH=CH–CH($OSiMe_2Bu^t$)–C_5H_{11})

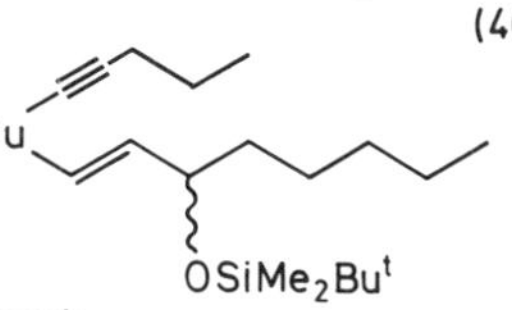

(*d*) HCl, H_2O, $(CH_3)_2CO$; (*e*) chromatography.

Figure 9.13: Synthesis of 10,11-trimethylene-11-deoxy PGE_1 methyl ester

No activity has been reported for the methylene and ethylene analogues (34) and (37), but the trimethylene compound (40) is reported to have thromboxane-like activity.

Ring fusion across the 11- and 12-positions has also been studied[15]. Thus, the 11,12-difluoromethylene analogues (41) and (42) have been prepared.

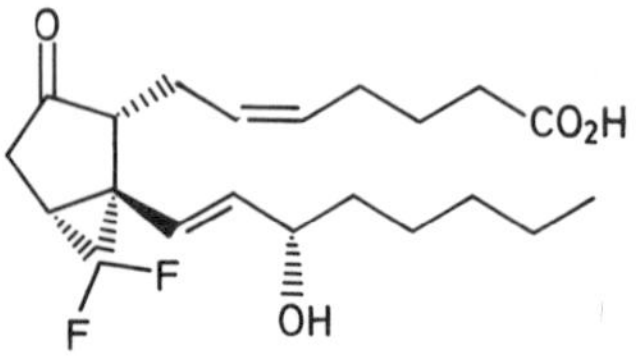

(41)

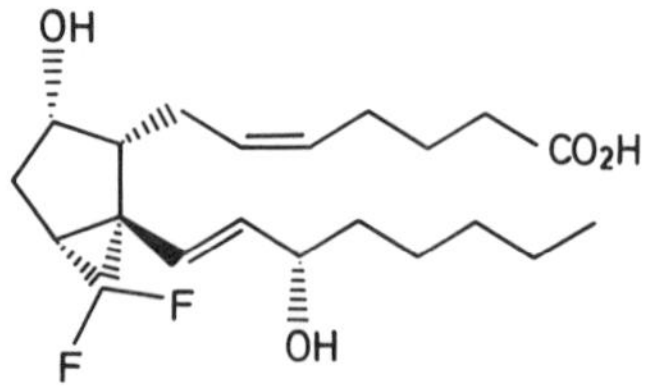

(42)

The compound (42) has 0.05 times the activity of PGE_2 as a bronchodilator after intravenous administration to guinea-pigs. Much greater activity, five times that of PGE_2, was shown by (41), but the compound was less active ($0.3 \times PGE_2$) after aerosol administration. Compound (41) has been examined as a bronchodilator in mildly asthmatic patients but has shown insufficient potency to be of interest[15].

Replacement of the cyclopentane ring

Many analogues are known in which the cyclopentane ring is replaced by other systems[17]. Several phenyl and substituted phenyl analogues are known but no significant activity was shown. The effect of replacement by both larger and smaller alicyclic rings has also been studied[17]. Cyclohexane analogues of PGE_2 (43) and $PGF_{2\alpha}$ (44) have been synthesized but were less active than the natural prostaglandins in a number of biological assays.

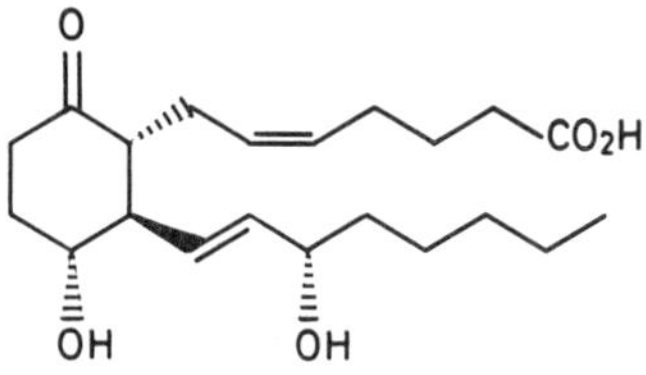

(43)

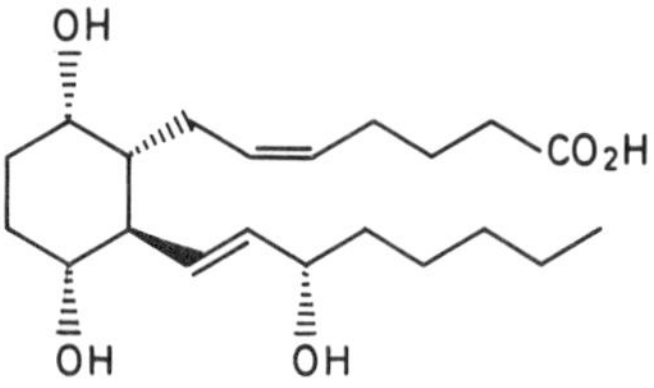

(44)

The cyclobutane analogues (47) and (48) have been prepared from the cycloadduct of cyclopentadiene and dichloroketene (45), which was transformed as shown in *Figure 9.14* into the lactone (46). This was converted into the products (47) and (48) using standard methods. No activity has been reported for either compound.

Considerable interest has been shown in replacing the cyclopentane ring with heterocyclic systems[7, 17, 19]. Several analogues have been prepared based on aromatic heterocyclic systems such as furan, pyrrole, oxazole, thiazole,

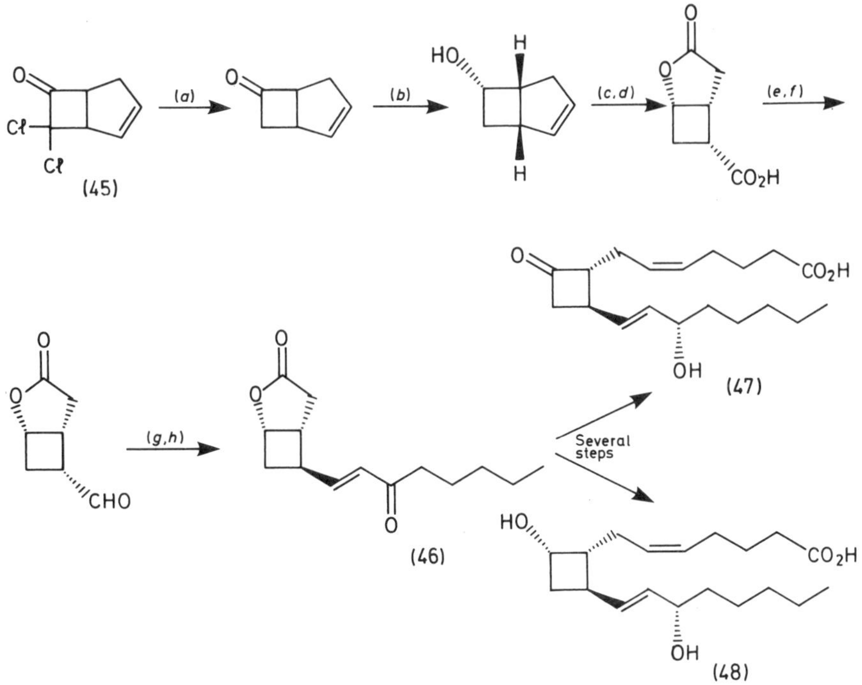

Reagents :- (*a*) Zn, AcOH ; (*b*) $LiAlH_4$; (*c*) O_3; (*d*) H_2O_2, HCO_2H ; (*e*) B_2H_6 ;
(*f*) pyridinium chlorochromate ; (*g*) dimethyl 2-oxoheptylphosphonate ;
(*h*) equilibration using 1,5-diazabicyclo[5.4.0]undec-5-ene.

Figure 9.14: Synthesis of cyclobutane analogues of PGs

imidazole, and indole, but where any prostaglandin-like activity has been reported it was generally weak. Greater interest has been shown in the synthesis of compounds containing saturated heterocyclic systems.

11-Deoxy-11-oxa-PGE_1 (49) has been synthesized and is reported to stimulate gerbil colon with a potency of 0.05 to 0.005 times that of PGE_2.

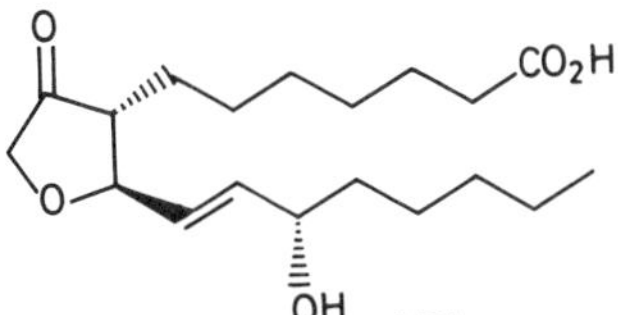

The 11-thia analogues (50) and (51) have also been prepared and both compounds have similar activity to (49).

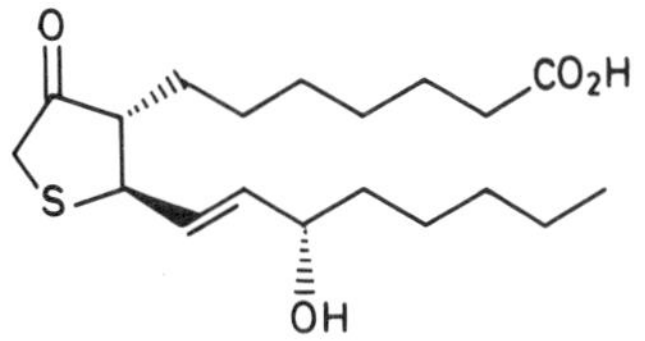

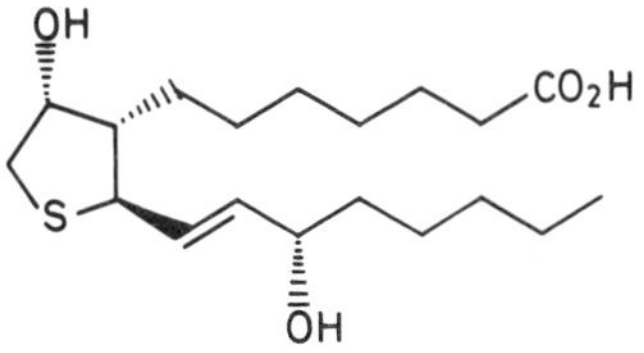

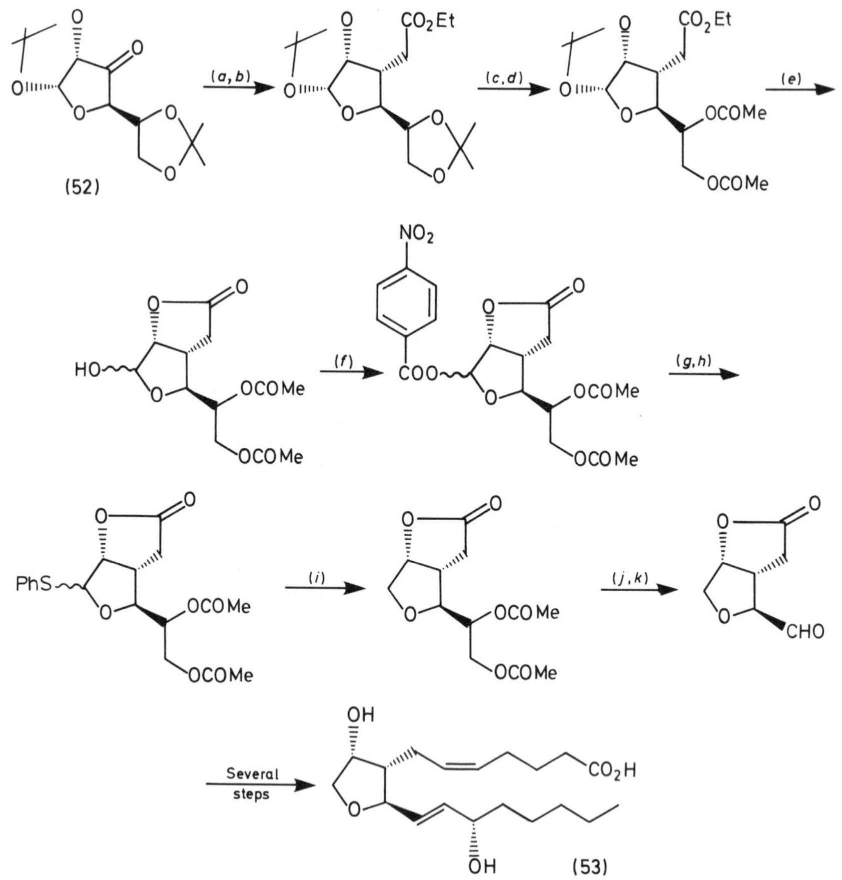

(52)

(53)

Reagents: (*a*) diethyl phosphonoacetate; (*b*) H_2, Ni; (*c*) AcOH, H_2O, 70 °C; (*d*) Ac_2O, C_5H_5N; (*e*) 80% AcOH; 90 °C; (*f*) *p*-nitrobenzoyl chloride, C_5H_5N; (*g*) HBr, $CHCl_3$, (*h*) potassium thiophenoxide, EtOH; (*i*) Raney Ni; (*j*) K_2CO_3, MeOH, H_2O; (*k*) $NaIO_4$.

Figure 9.15: Synthesis of 11-deoxy-11-oxa $PGF_{2\alpha}$

9-Deoxy-9-oxaprostaglandins and some thia analogues have also been prepared but nothing is known of their biological properties.

Both 11-deoxy-11-oxa-PGE_2 and 11-deoxy-11-oxa-$PGF_{2\alpha}$ (53) have been prepared. An interesting synthesis of the latter compound is that of Lourens and Koekemoer (*see Figure 9.15*), in which a simple derivative of D-glucose (52) is converted into (53) with control of stereochemistry at all chiral centres.

Azaprostaglandins are known with a nitrogen atom in all possible positions of the ring but greatest interest has centred on 8- and 12-aza analogues.

Several groups have reported syntheses of 8-azaprostaglandins but in all cases the synthetic strategy is similar, the starting material being a

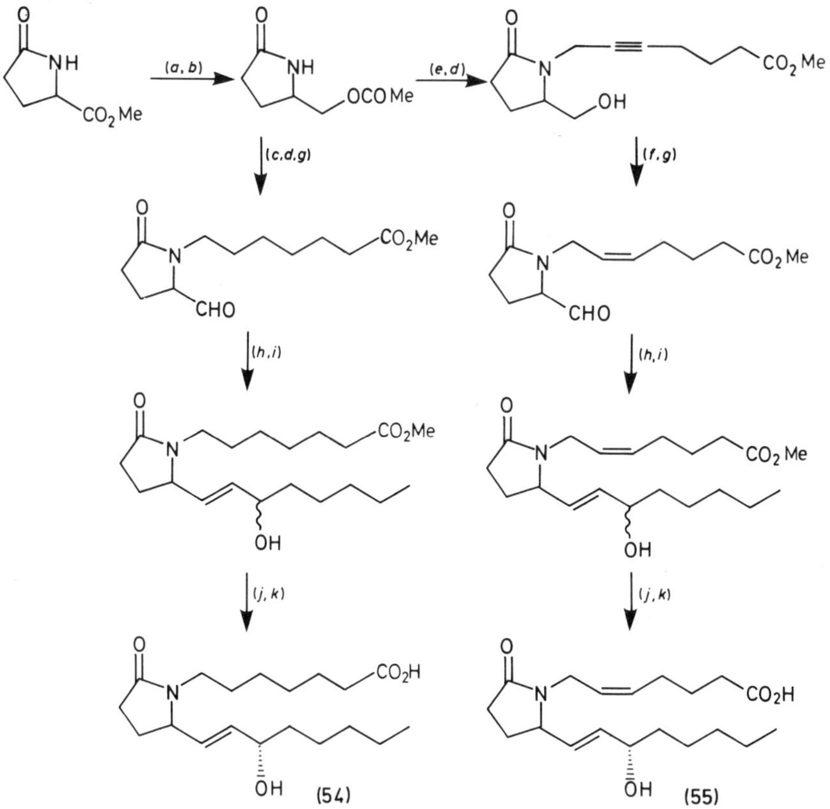

Reagents :- (a) $LiBH_4$; (b) Ac_2O, C_5H_5N; (c) NaH, $Br(CH_2)_6CO_2Me$, KI, DMF; (d) K_2CO_3, MeOH; (e) methyl 7-bromohept-5-ynoate; (f) H_2, Pd, $BaSO_4$; (g) dicyclohexylcarbodi-imide, DMSO; (h) dimethyl 2-oxoheptyl-phosphonate; (i) $Zn(BH_4)_2$; (j) chromatography to separate C-15 epimers; (k) KOH, EtOH, H_2O.

Figure 9.16: Synthesis of 8-aza-11-deoxy PGEs

pyroglutamic acid derivative. The synthesis of de Koning and co-workers (*see Figure 9.16*) is typical.

The acids (54) and (55) were both found to be substrates for 15-hydroxy-prostaglandin dehydrogenase. The methyl ester precursor or (54) is claimed to lower blood pressure and inhibit gastric ulcer formation.

Several 12-azaprostaglandins are known, the most interesting being the compound (56), incorporating the pyrrolidine-2,4-dione system[20].

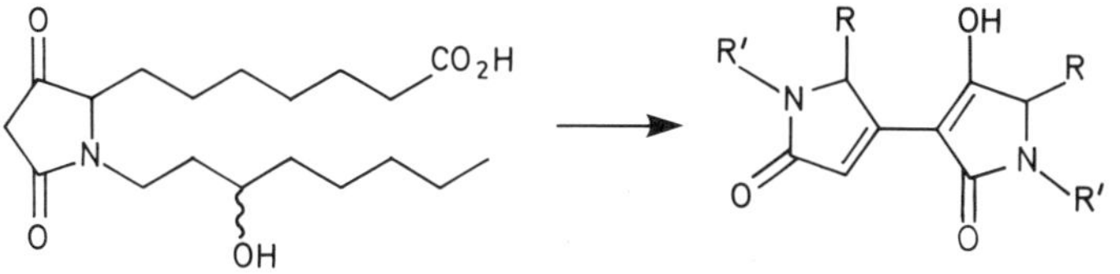

(56) (57)

It was found that the pyrrolidinedione system of (56) underwent a ready intermolecular condensation to give an anhydro-dimer of the type (57). Because of this, chromatographic separation of the diastereomeric mixture of acids (56) was not possible. Nevertheless, the mixture was found to have a profile of activity qualitatively similar to that of PGE_2 on a variety of smooth muscle preparations although it was about 1000 times less potent. It was also shown to be a moderately potent inhibitor of platelet aggregation and lowered blood pressure in rats after intravenous administration. Although (56) was less active than PGE_2, it was found to have the advantage of not being removed during passage through the pulmonary circulation.

The activity of (56) was followed up by the synthesis of related structures in which anhydro-dimer formation cannot occur. The hydantoin derivative (58) was prepared as shown in *Figure 9.17*[21].

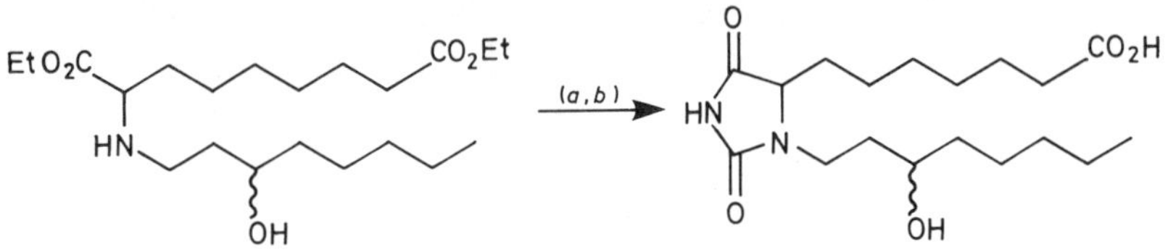

Reagents: (*a*) HCNO, heat ; (*b*) NaOH , H_2O.

Figure 9.17: Preparation of the hydantoin (58)

The diastereomeric mixture of acids (58) was separated by chromatography and the less polar diastereoisomer was found to be about twice as active as PGE_1 as an inhibitor of platelet aggregation. In a structure-activity study it was found that replacing the terminal n-pentyl by cycloalkyl groups increased activity further. The most active compound was the cyclohexyl analogue (59), which was 14 times more potent as an inhibitor of platelet aggregation than PGE_1, but was less active as a vasodilator. The activity was shown to reside in the enantiomer with the absolute configuration as indicated.

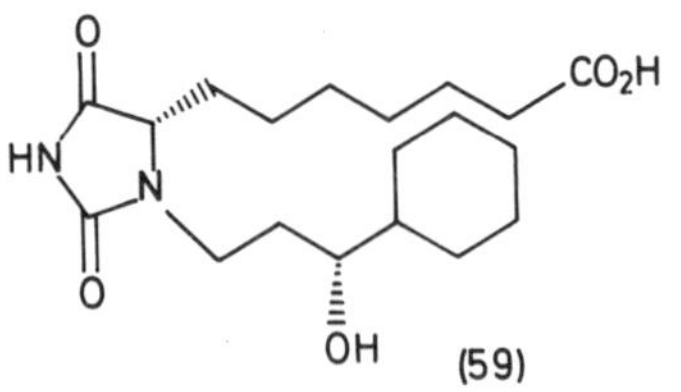

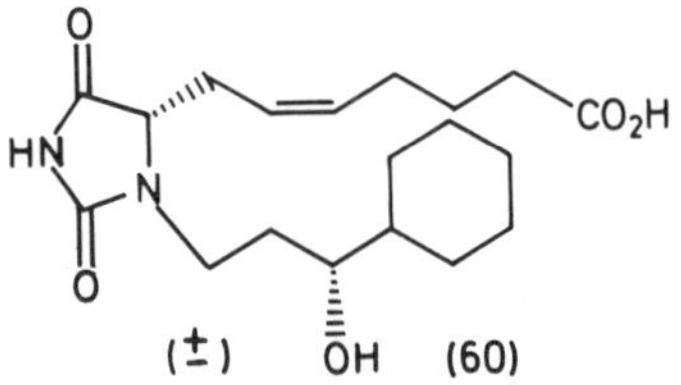

The 5,6-dehydro analogue (60) was prepared by a similar route and the less polar diastereoisomer was shown to be about 22 times more potent that PGE_1 as a platelet aggregation inhibitor. Moreover, it had virtually no effect on intestinal smooth muscle and caused less vasodilatation than PGE_1.

Compounds with the profile of activity shown by (59) and (60) have potential as antithrombotic drugs.

Prostaglandin endoperoxide analogues

The discovery that prostaglandin endoperoxides, in addition to being precursors of the prostaglandins, are very potent constrictors of smooth muscle and cause platelet aggregation, has stimulated interest in the synthesis of analogues in which the labile peroxy bridge is replaced by more stable units[22]. The elucidation of the thromboxane pathway from PGH_2 has added additional impetus to synthesis in this area, since a close analogue of PGH_2 might be expected to inhibit the thromboxane synthetase enzyme thereby preventing the formation of TXA_2. An inhibitor of TXA_2 synthetase, which lacks PGH_2-like activity, is potentially of great value for the treatment of cardiovascular conditions where vasospasm or platelet aggregation are thought to play a major role, such as angina, heart attack, stroke, etc.

The endoperoxide analogue (61) in which the peroxy linkage is replaced by an ethylenic double bond has been prepared by Corey and co-workers using the Diels-Alder adduct of cyclopentadiene and methyl propiolate as the starting material (*see Figure 9.18*).

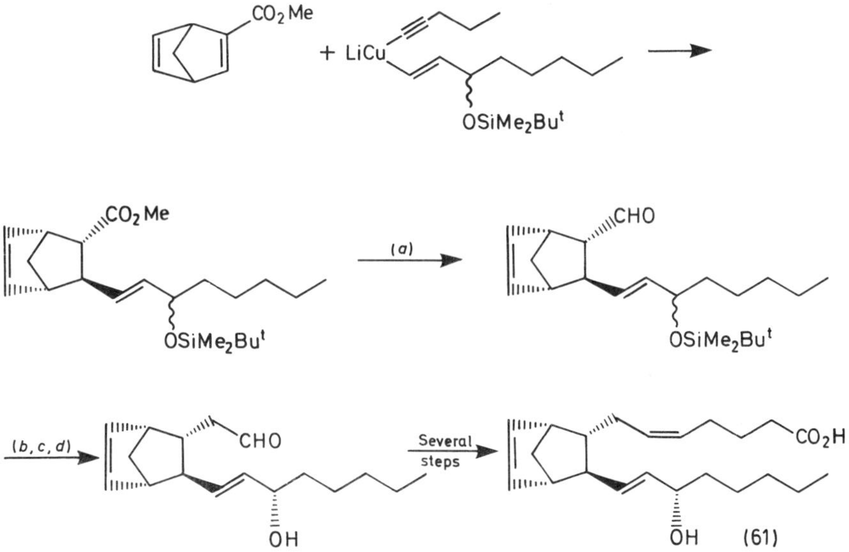

Reagents; (*a*) di-isobutylaluminium hydride, CH_2Cl_2;
(*b*) methoxymethylenetriphenylphosphorane, toluene, THF;
(*c*) AcOH, THF, H_2O; (*d*) chromatography to separate C–15 OH epimers.

Figure 9.18: Synthesis of the bicyclo[2.2.1]hept-2-ene (61)

The product (61) was about 10 times less active than PGG_2 in causing aggregation in human platelet-rich plasma.

Most of the other endoperoxide analogues reported contain one or more heteroatoms in the 9,11-linkage and, in nearly all cases, synthesis has been carried out by modification of a derivative of a natural prostaglandin.

Bundy[14] has reported the synthesis of compounds in which either oxygen

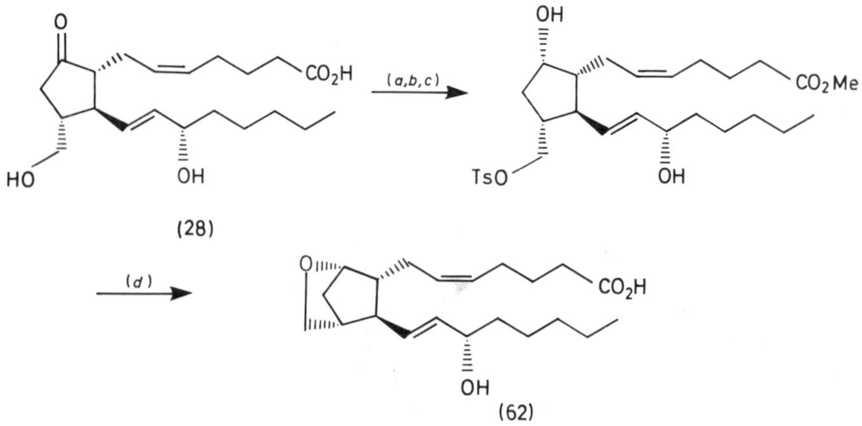

(28)

(62)

Reagents:-(*a*) lithium perhydro-9b-boraphenalyl hydride; (*b*) diazomethane; (*c*) *p*-toluenesulphonyl (Ts) chloride, C_5H_5N; (*d*) KOH, MeOH, H_2O.

Figure 9.19: Synthesis of 9,11-epoxymethano-PG (62)

of the peroxy linkage of PGH_2 is replaced by a methylene unit. The 9,11-epoxymethano analogue (62) was prepared as outlined in *Figure 9.19*.

The 11,9-epoxymethano isomer (67) was synthesized using the PGE_2 derivative (63) as starting material and was found to be 6.2 times more active than PGH_2 in causing contraction of isolated rabbit aorta and 3.2 times more active than PGG_2 in causing aggregation of human platelets. The 9,11-epoxymethano isomer (62) was less active in these test systems. Both isomers have been reported to inhibit thromboxane synthetase, (62) being about 20 times more potent than (64)[23].

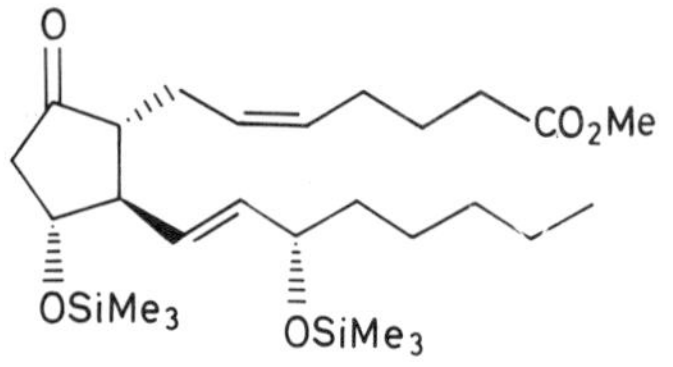

(63)

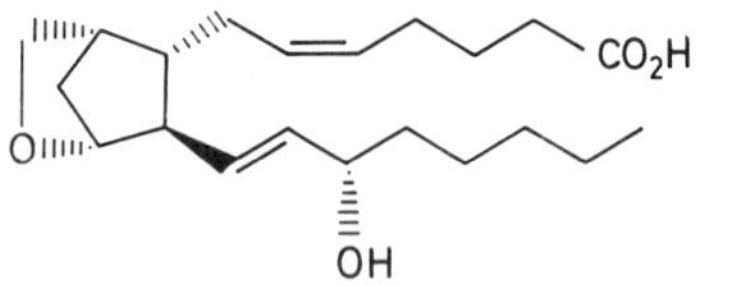

(64)

Corey and Niwa[24] have reported the synthesis of the cyclic amine derivatives (65) by the route shown (*see Figure 9.20*).

The product (65) was found to be a potent inhibitor of thromboxane synthetase but its endoperoxide-like activity has not been reported.

Other endoperoxide analogues are known which contain two heteroatoms in the 9,11-bridge. One of the most extensively studied compounds of this type is the 9,11-azo analogue (66) synthesized by Corey and co-workers (*see Figure 9.21*)[22].

The azo analogue (66) was 8 times more potent than PGG_2 in causing aggregation of human platelets and was about 7 times more potent than PGH_2 in causing contraction of isolated rabbit aorta. It was also found to be

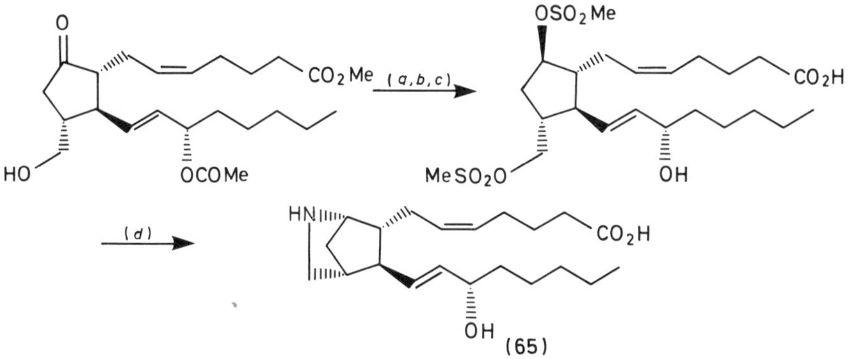

(65)

Reagents: (*a*) $NaBH_4$; (*b*) $MeSO_2Cl$, $(C_2H_5)_3N$, CH_2Cl_2; (*c*) LiOH, MeOH; (*d*) NH_4OH.

Figure 9.20: Preparation of PG-analogue (65)

a potent inhibitor of thromboxane synthetase, being about 10 times more potent than the 9,11-epoxymethano analogue (62). It is also a potent inhibitor of PGI_2 synthetase[24].

Hayashi and co-workers have prepared the 9,11-dithia analogue of PGH_2 (67) by the route outlined in *Figure 9.22*[22].

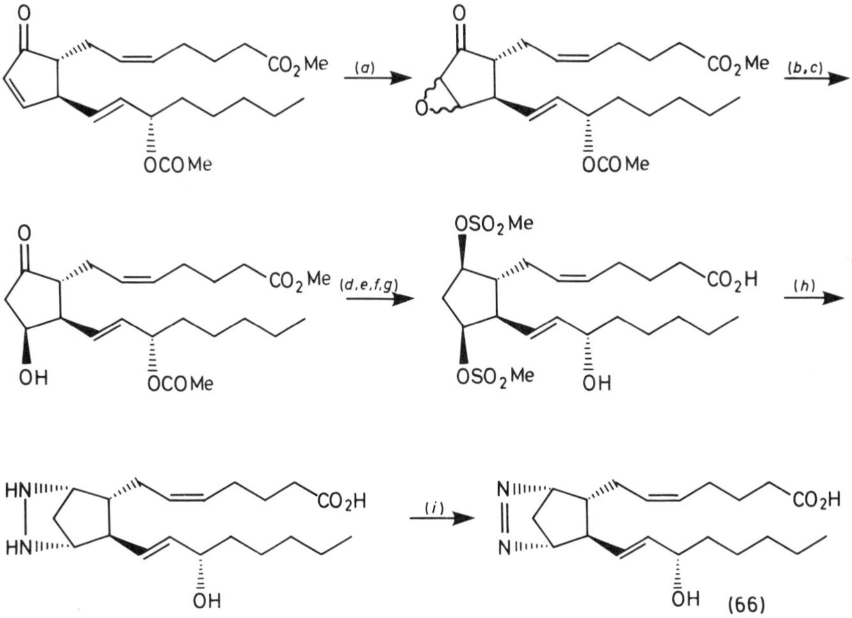

(66)

Reagents:- (*a*) H_2O_2, MeOH, NaOH; (*b*) Al/Hg, THF, H_2O; (*c*) chromatography; (*d*) $Zn(BH_4)_2$; (*e*) $MeSO_2Cl$, Et_3N, CH_2Cl_2; (*f*) chromatography; (*g*) LiOH, MeOH, H_2O; (*h*) N_2H_4; (*i*) Air, $Cu(OCOMe)_2$, MeOH, ether.

Figure 9.21: Synthesis of the 9,11-azo analogue of PGH_2

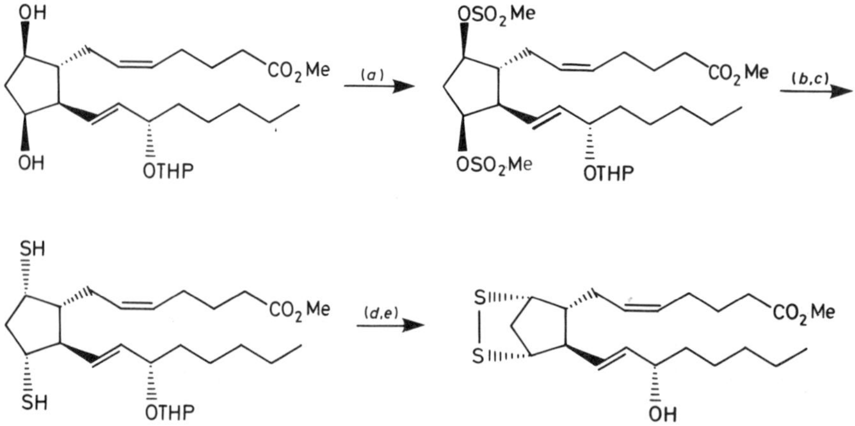

(67)

Reagents: (*a*) $MeSO_2Cl$, Et_3N, CH_2Cl_2 ; (*b*) AcSNa, DMF, DMSO ; (*c*) K_2CO_3, MeOH ; (*d*) MnO_2, toluene ; (*e*) AcOH, THF, H_2O.

Figure 9.22: Synthesis of the 9,11-dithia analogue of PGH_2

The endosulphide (67) had aorta-contracting activity 24 times greater than that of PGH_2 and also caused rapid and irreversible aggregation of human platelets.

Although several of the endoperoxide analogues mentioned above block the formation of TXA_2 from PGH_2, most have also been reported to have endoperoxide and TXA_2-like activity in their own right and thus have no potential utility as antithrombotic drugs. However, an important observation in this connection was made by workers at the Upjohn Company, who found that the analogue of the azo compound (66) lacking a hydroxyl group at C-15, (68), was practically devoid of endoperoxide-like activity but was still a potent TXA_2 synthetase inhibitor[26].

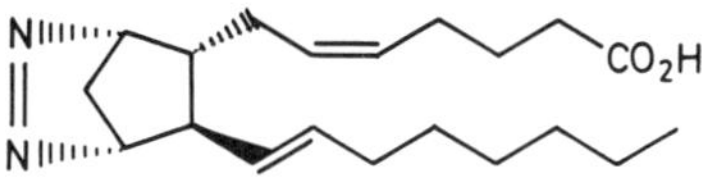

(68)

Unfortunately (68), like (66), is a potent inhibitor of PGI_2 formation from PGH_2[25]. Since PGI_2 is a potent vasodilator and inhibitor of platelet aggregation, inhibition of its synthesis is clearly undesirable in an antithrombotic agent.

The Upjohn group have also reported the synthesis of 15-deoxy analogues containing an epoxyimino linkage, for example (69).

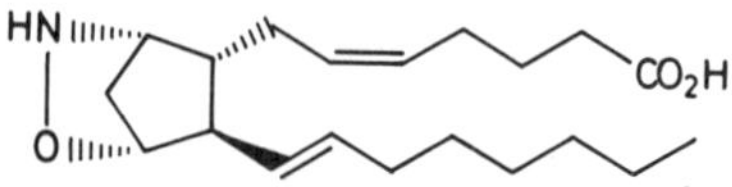

(69)

This compound was almost as potent a TXA_2 synthetase inhibitor as the azo analogue (68), but had no effect on PGI_2 synthetase. In fact in rabbit lung microsomes which contain both TXA_2 and PGI_2 synthetases, the decrease in TXA_2 formation produced by (69) was accompanied by an increase in PGI_2 production, resulting from diversion of the endoperoxide substrate to the PGI_2 pathway[27]. A compound capable of causing this effect *in vivo* could be useful in treating conditions in which the balance between TXA_2 and PGI_2 is altered in favour of the former.

Prostaglandin I_2 analogues

The discovery of PGI_2 and its potent vasodilator and platelet aggregation inhibitory actions has stimulated great interest in the synthesis of analogues as potential antithrombotic agents[22]. The inherent acid instability of PGI_2 due to its enol ether linkage imposes a severe limitation on its clinical use, although PGI_2 infusion has some potential in the prevention of platelet

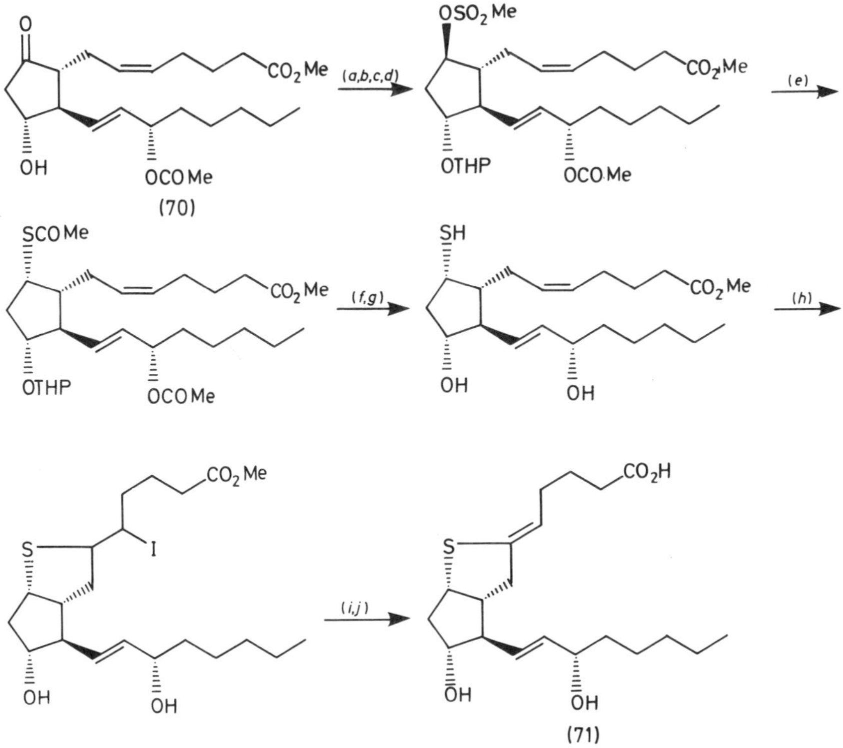

Reagents: (*a*) dihydropyran, H^+, CH_2Cl_2; (*b*) $Zn(BH_4)_2$; (*c*) chromatography to remove 9α-epimer; (*d*) CH_3SO_2Cl, $(C_2H_5)_3N$, CH_2Cl_2; (*e*) CH_3COSK, DMSO; (*f*) CH_3CO_2H, THF, H_2O; (*g*) K_2CO_3, CH_3OH; (*h*) I_2, K_2CO_3, CH_2Cl_2; (*i*) 1,5-diazabicyclo [5.4.0] undec-5-ene, C_6H_6; (*j*) C_2H_5ONa, C_2H_5OH.

Figure 9.23: Synthesis of 6,9-thia-PGI_2

aggregation during cardiopulmonary bypass and haemodialysis. However, for more general use, an orally active analogue is a desirable goal and much of the synthetic work in this area has centred on replacement of the labile enol ether linkage with more stable units.

Nicolaou and co-workers[28] have reported the synthesis of the sulphur analogue of PGI_2 (71) starting from the PGE_2 derivative (70) (*see Figure 9.23*).

The thia analogue (71) shows PGI_2-like relaxant activity on bovine coronary artery and is also a potent inhibitor of platelet aggregation with a potency of 0.04 to 0.5 times that of PGI_2, depending on the test system used. Surprisingly, however, (71) also exhibits some thromboxane-like activity in that it is a potent constrictor of cat coronary artery and rabbit mesenteric artery. In an *in vivo* model for measuring platelet aggregation in cats, the disaggregatory activity of (71) was 10 to 20 times less than that of PGI_2 and the duration of action was no longer. Since (71) has greater chemical stability than PGI_2, the poor duration of action suggests that rapid metabolism may be occurring[28, 29].

The sulphoxide and sulphone derivatives (72) and (73) had little or no effect on platelet aggregation or cat coronary artery[28].

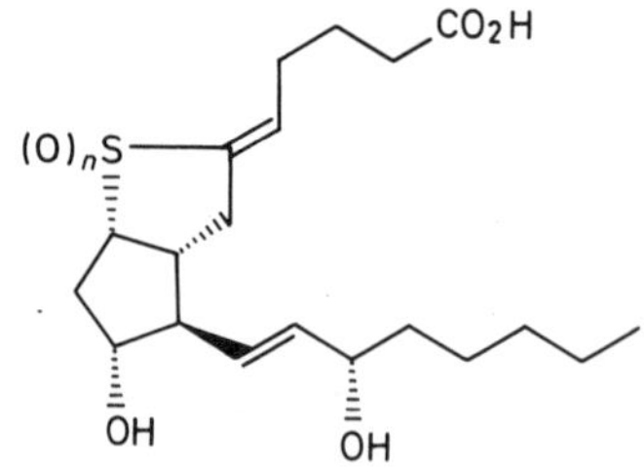

(72) $n=1$

(73) $n=2$

Several groups have reported the synthesis of the analogue (75), in which the ether linkage is replaced by a methylene unit. Japanese workers have reported a synthesis from the optically active lactone (74), which is readily available from the work of Corey (*see* Chapter 4)[30].

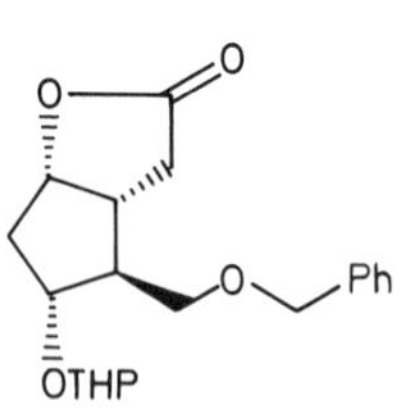

(74) 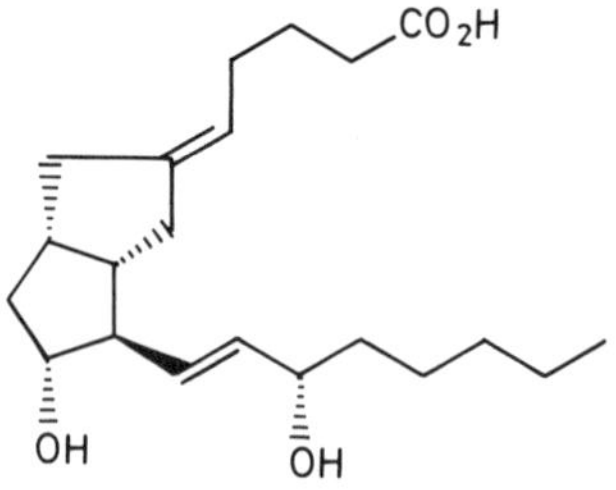 (75)

The methylene analogue (75) was found to have a potency of 0.03 times that of PGI_2 as an inhibitor of aggregation of human, dog and rabbit platelets. In *in vivo* models of platelet aggregation in dogs and rabbits it had 0.1 times the activity of PGI_2. It causes a reduction in systemic arterial blood pressure in dogs, rabbits and rats after intravenous administration. It is also a potent inhibitor of gastric acid secretion in rats after intravenous infusion, having 0.4 times the activity of PGI_2[31, 32].

Unfortunately, like the thia analogue (71), (75) has a duration of action *in vivo* no greater than that of PGI_2, again suggesting rapid metabolism. The compound does not appear to be deactivated by passage through the lungs in rats, but it has been found to be a substrate for the 15-hydroxyprostaglandin dehydrogenase enzyme[31, 32].

Nitrogen-containing analogues have been prepared by Upjohn workers. The analogue (77) was prepared from the $PGF_{2\alpha}$ derivative (76) as shown in *Figure 9.24*[33].

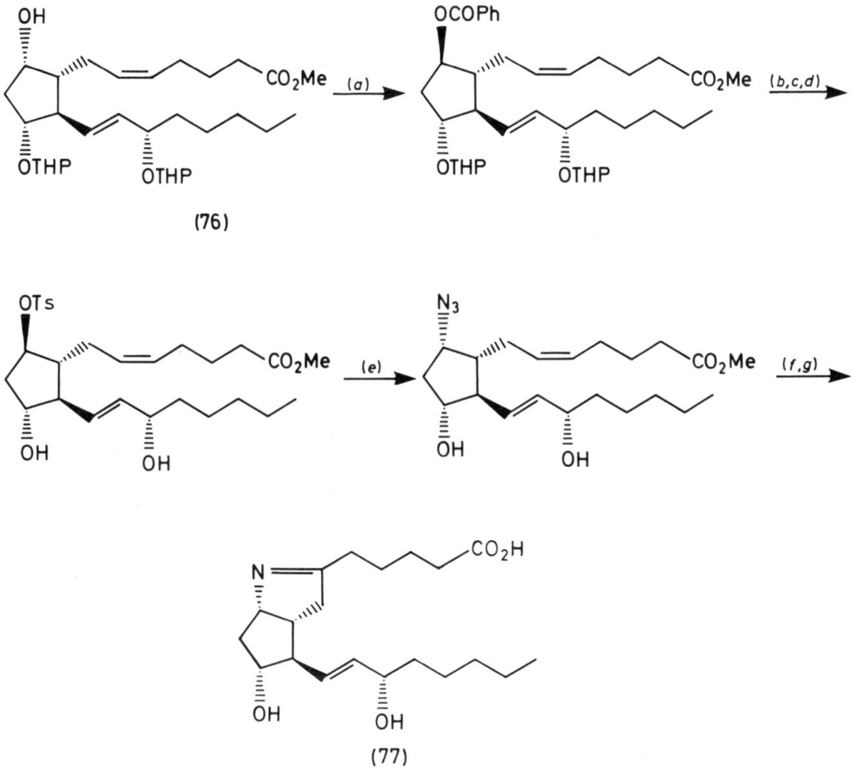

Reagents:- (*a*) $PhCO_2H$, Ph_3P, diethyl azodicarboxylate; (*b*) MeONa, MeOH; (*c*) *p*-toluenesulphonyl chloride, C_5H_5N; (*d*) $MeCO_2H$, THF, H_2O; (*e*) NaN_3, hexamethylphosphoramide; (*f*) heat 70 – 80 °C; (*g*) OH^-.

Figure 9.24: Synthesis of the aza-analogue (77) of PGI_2

Antiaggregatory activity approaching that of PGI_2 was shown by (77), but the compound was considerably less active as a vasodepressor in the cat. The dihydro compounds (78) and (79), obtained by reduction of the ester precursor of (77) followed by hydrolysis, were found to be only very weak inhibitors of platelet aggregation.

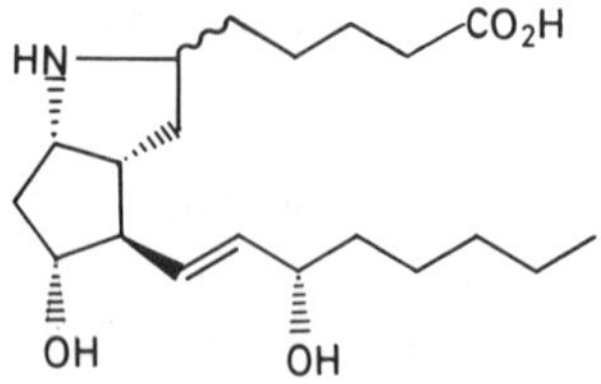

(78) 6α

(79) 6β

Continued synthetic effort can be expected in this area in the future. However, from the initial results obtained with the first stable PGI_2 analogues, it is already apparent that chemical stability alone may be insufficient to guarantee the desired duration of action *in vivo* and that metabolic stability will also have to be achieved.

References

1. A. HAMON, B. LACOUME, G. PASQUET and W.R. PILGRIM, *Tetrahedron Lett.*, 1976, 211.
2. E.J. COREY, C.S. SHINER, R.P. VOLANTE and C.R. CYR, *Tetrahedron Lett.*, 1975, 1161.
3. E.J. COREY and M.S. SACHDEV, *J. Am. chem. Soc.*, 1973, **95,** 8483.
4. S.M. ROBERTS and F. SCHEINMANN (Ed), *Chemistry, Biochemistry and Pharmacological Activity of Prostanoids,* Pergamon Press, 1979, p 87.
5. P.A. GRIECO, W. OWENS, C-L.J. WANG, E. WILLIAMS, W.J. SCHILLINGER, K. HIROTSU and J. CLARDY, *J. med. Chem.*, 1980, **23,** 1072.
6. J.S. BINDRA and R. BINDRA, *Prostaglandin Synthesis,* Academic Press, 1977, Chapter 20.
7. A. MITRA, *The Synthesis of Prostaglandins,* John Wiley & Sons, 1977. Chapter 19.
8. M.E. ROSENTHALE, A. DERVINIS and D. STRIKE in *Adv. Prostaglandin and Thromboxane Res.*, Raven Press, 1976, **1,** 477.
9. M.P.L. CATON and K. CROWSHAW, in *Prog. med. Chem.*, North Holland Publishing Co., **15,** 357.
10. L.A. HOHNKE, J.F. EGGLER and J.N. PEREIRA, *Absts., 4th Int. Prostaglandin Conference,* Washington D.C., 1979, 49.
11. N. FINCH, J.J. FITT and I.H.S. HSU, *J. org. Chem.*, 1975, **40,**
12. C.V. GRUDZINSKAS and M. WEISS, *Tetrahedron Lett.*, 1973, 141.
13. M.B. FLOYD, R.E. SCHAUB, G.J. SIUTA, J.S. SKOTNICKI, C.V. GRUDZINSKAS, M.J. WEISS, F. DESSY and L. VANHUMBEECK, *J. med. Chem.*, 1980, **23,** 903.
14. G.L. BUNDY, *Tetrahedron Lett.*, 1975, 1957.
15. *Ref. 4*, p. 39.
16. O. ODA, K. KOKIMA and K. SAKAI, *Tetrahedron Lett.*, 1975, 3705 and 3709.
17. *Ref. 6,* Chapter 21.
18. R.F. NEWTON, P.L. PAUSON and R.G. TAYLOR, *J. chem. Res.*, 1980, (S) 277.
19. D. ORTH and H-E RADUNZ, *Top. Curr. Chem.*, 1977, **72,** 51.
20. C.J. HARRIS, N. WHITTAKER, G.A. HIGGS, J.M. ARMSTRONG and P.M. REED, *Prostaglandins,* 1978, **16,** 773.
21. A.G. CALDWELL, *et al., J.C.S. Chem. Comm.*, 1979, 561; *J. Chem. Soc., Perkin Trans. I,* 1980, 495.
22. K.C. NICOLAOU, G.P. GASIC and W.E. BARNETTE, *Angew. Chem. Int. Ed.*, 1978, **17,** 293.
23. F.F. SUN, *Biochem. biophys. Res. Commun.*, 1977, **74,** 1432.
24. E.J. COREY, M. NIWA, M. BLOOM and P.W. RAMWELL, *Tetrahedron Lett.*, 1979, 671.
25. D.P. WALLACH, *Prostaglandins,* 1978, **15,** 671.
26. *Ref. 4,* p. 115.

27. F. FITZPATRICK, R. GORMAN, G. BUNDY, R. HONOHAN, J. McGUIRE AND F. SUN, *Biochim. biophys. Acta,* 1979, **573,** 238.
28. *Ref. 4,* p. 286.
29. R.J. GRYGLEWSKI, K.C. NICOLAOU, *Experientia,* 1978, **34,** 1336.
30. Y. KONISHI, M. KAWAMURA, Y. ARAI and M. HAYASHI, *Chem. Lett.,* 1979, 1437.
31. B.J.R. WHITTLE, S. MONCADA, F. WHITING and J.R. VANE, *Prostaglandins,* 1980, **19,** 605.
32. J.W. AIKEN and R.J. SHEBUSKI, *Prostaglandins,* 1980, **19,** 629.
33. G.L. BUNDY and J.M. BALDWIN, *Tetrahedron Lett.,* 1978, 1371.

CHAPTER 10

Synthesis and biological activity of thromboxane A_2 (TXA_2) analogues

Richard J.K. Taylor
School of Chemical Sciences, University of East Anglia, Norwich, Norfolk

Introduction

The biological potency of TXA_2 combined with its short biological half life stimulated the search for stable synthetic analogues. Stable TXA_2 analogues would help to evaluate the biological role of the parent compound and may prove to be of therapeutic value. A stable TXA_2 analogue, which antagonizes the action of TXA_2 itself, would have potential application in the treatment of cardiovascular complaints such as thrombosis. The instability of TXA_2 is due to the dioxabicyclo[3.1.1]heptane system; hydrolysis of the bicyclic acetal to give TXB_2 releases the strain associated with the four-membered oxetane ring.

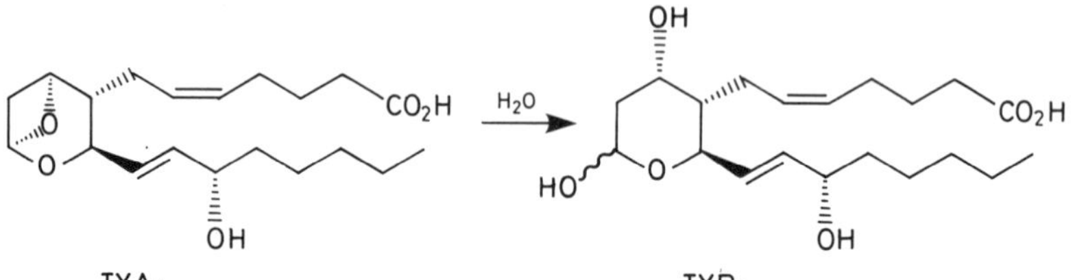

OH CO2H H2O CO2H HO O O O OH OH

TXA_2 TXB_2

Structural analogues of TXA_2 in which one or both oxygen atoms are replaced by methylene groups would be expected to be far more resistant to hydrolysis. This hypothesis has been confirmed as can be seen from the following discussion.

TXA_2 ether analogues

Both of the possible bicyclic ether analogues of TXA_2 (1) and (2) have been prepared. A group from the Upjohn Company prepared 11a-carba-TXA_2 (1), which apparently inhibits the aggregation of human platelets[1]. E.J.

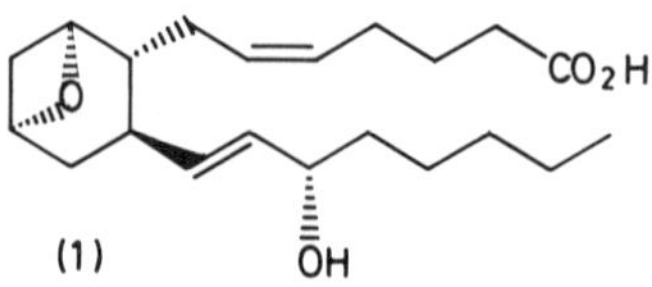

O CO2H OH (1) CO2H O OH (2)

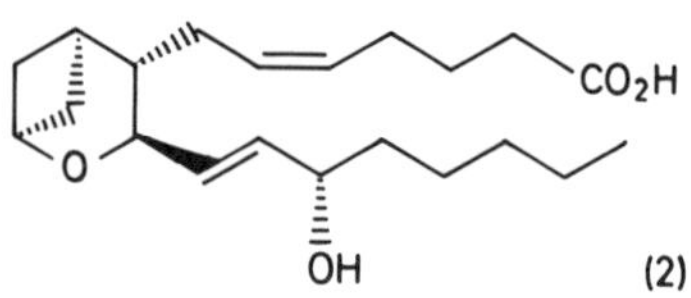

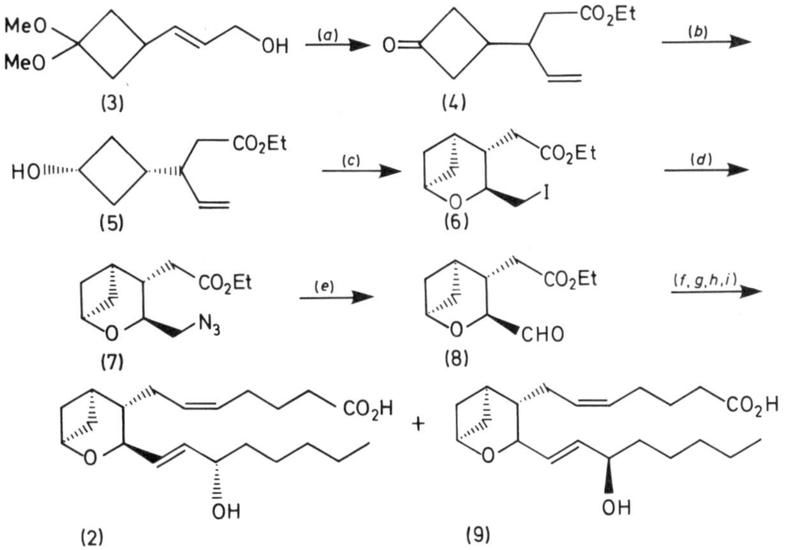

(3) (4) (5) (6) (7) (8) (2) (9)

Reagents:- (*a*) $(EtO)_3CMe$, $EtCO_2H$, 142 °C then 1M HCl (*ca.* 74%); (*b*) $NaBH_4$, EtOH, −60 °C (96%); (*c*) $Hg(OCOCF_3)_2$, benzene, 23 °C then I_2 (40%); (*d*) NaN_3, DMF, 100 °C (80%); (*e*) FSO_3Me, 23 °C; (*f*) $(MeO)_2P(O)\overset{-}{C}HC(O)C_5H_{11}\overset{+}{Na}$; (*g*) $Zn(BH_4)_2$, DME, 23 °C; (*h*) Bu^i_2AlH; (*i*) $Ph_3P{=}CH(CH_2)_3CO_2Na$, DMSO.

Figure 10.1: Synthesis of TXA_2 analogue (2)

Corey and his co-workers prepared the analogue (2), in which a methylene group replaces the 9,11-bridging oxygen of TXA_2, by the synthetic route shown in *Figure 10.1*[2].

The protected 3-substituted cyclobutanone (3) was prepared from *trans*-2,4-pentadien-1-ol in five steps (silylation, dichloroketene addition, dechlorination, desilylation and acetal formation). On heating with triethyl orthoacetate, (3) gave (4) by way of a Claisen rearrangement, acetal hydrolysis also occurring during this reaction. Reduction of (4) with sodium borohydride took place from the least hindered face of the molecule giving the alcohol (5) stereospecifically.

The key step in this synthesis was the stereospecific intramolecular cyclization of (5) to give the bicylic compound (6). After a great deal of experimentation, this cyclization was achieved using the oxymercuration reaction, followed by replacement of mercury by iodine.

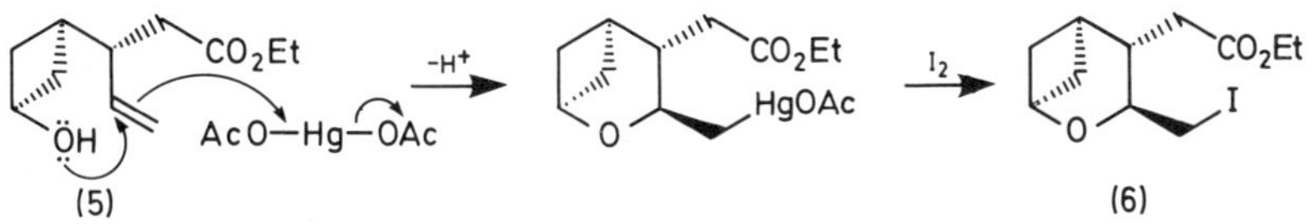

(5) AcO—Hg—OAc $-H^+$ HgOAc I_2 (6)

Molecular models indicate that the preferred mode of cyclization leads to a *trans*-relationship between the side chains and this was observed in practice.

Problems were encountered when the conversion of iodide (6) into aldehyde (8) was attempted using standard procedures. These difficulties were overcome by devising a novel method for carrying out this transformation. Iodide (6) was converted into azide (7) which gave the required aldehyde (8) when treated with methylfluorosulphonate.

The synthesis was then completed using standard prostaglandin reactions giving TXA_2 analogue (2) along with its 15β-epimer (9). Compounds (2) and (9) are reported to show interesting biological activities but full details have not yet been published.

Carbocyclic TXA_2 analogues

Two syntheses of carbocyclic-TXA_2 (10) have been published. The first was by Hiyashi and his colleagues from the Ono Pharmaceutical Company in

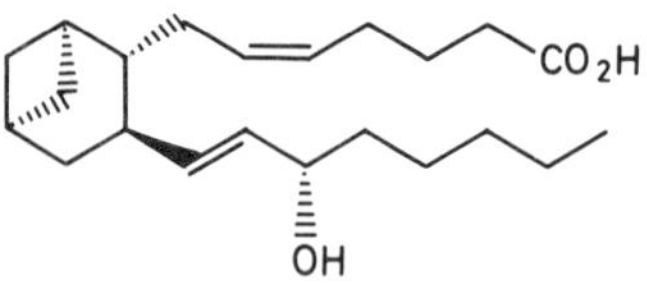

CO_2H
OH
(10)

Japan[3] and the second, by Nicolaou's group from the University of Pennsylvania[4], is shown in *Figure 10.2.*

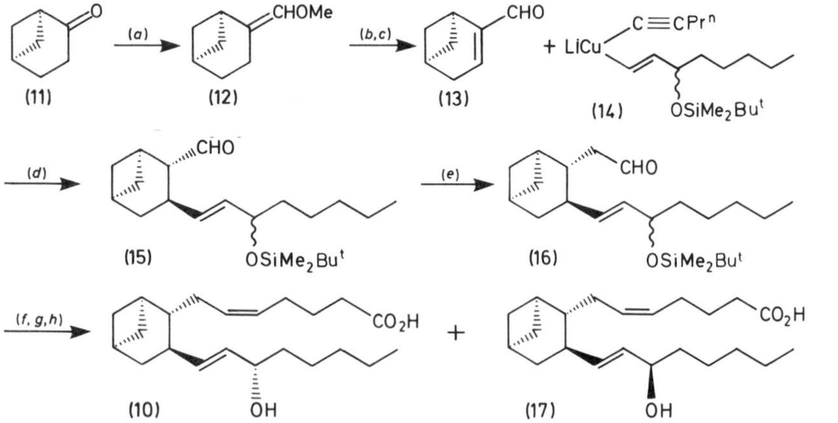

(11) → (a) → (12) CHOMe → (b,c) → (13) CHO + LiCu(C≡CPr^n) (14) OSiMe$_2$Bu^t

→ (d) → (15) CHO, OSiMe$_2$Bu^t → (e) → (16) CHO, OSiMe$_2$Bu^t

→ (f, g, h) → (10) CO_2H, OH + (17) CO_2H, OH

Reagents: (*a*) $Ph_3PCHOMe$, THF–toluene, 0 °C; (*b*) PhSeCl (excess), K_2CO_3, CH_2Cl_2–toluene, −78 °C; (*c*) MCPBA, CH_2Cl_2, −78 °C then Pr^i_2NH (55% from 12); (*d*) ether, −78 °C (53%); (*e*) $Ph_3PCHOMe$, toluene–THF, 0 °C then $Hg(OAc)_2$, H_2O–THF, 25 °C then 7% aq KI (79%); (*f*) $Ph_3PCH(CH_2)_3CO_2Na$, DMSO, 25 °C then CH_2N_2, 0 °C (74%); (*g*) AcOH–THF–H_2O (3:2:2), 45 °C then chromatography (65%, α-epimer, 33% β-epimer); (*h*) 1M LiOH, THF–H_2O (95–97%).

Figure 10.2: Synthesis of carbocyclic TXA_2

The bicyclic ketone (11) was converted into enol ether (12) using the Wittig reaction. Treatment of (12) with phenylselenyl chloride followed by peracid oxidation of the product gave the α,β-unsaturated aldehyde (13). This sequence exploits the electrophilicity of phenylselenyl chloride and the ease with which selenoxides undergo elimination.

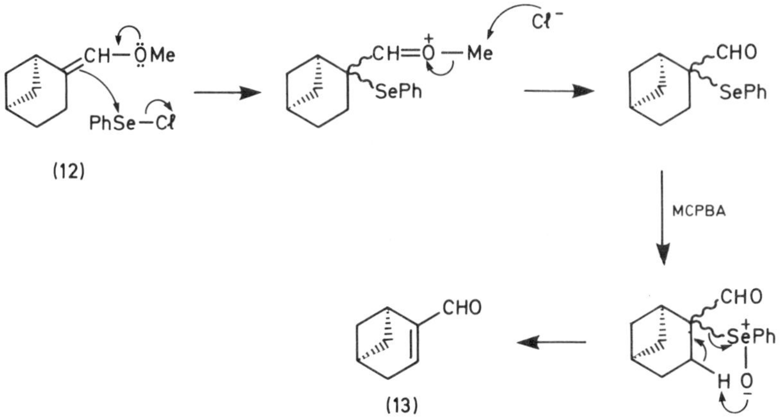

(12)

MCPBA

(13)

The key step in this synthesis involved the use of organocuprate reagent (14). Organocuprate reagents, R_2CuLi, generally give conjugate or 1,4-addition rather than 1,2-addition to α,β-unsaturated carbonyl compounds (*see* Chapter 5).

Thus, treatment of α,β-unsaturated aldehyde (13) with organocuprate (14) gave the desired adduct (15) in 53 per cent yield. Homologation of (15) using the Wittig reaction gave aldehyde (16), and completion of the synthesis using standard procedures gave carbocyclic TXA_2 (10) together with its 15β-epimer (17).

Carbocyclic TXA_2 (10) is stable and possesses extremely interesting biological properties. It mimics the behaviour of TXA_2 in its vasoconstricting ability[3,4], but it behaves as a potent TXA_2 antagonist in platelet aggregation assays[4]. Furthermore, analogue (10) selectively inhibits thromboxane biosynthesis without interfering with the production of prostacyclin[4].

Using similar procedures to those shown in *Figure 10.2*, Nicolaou's group prepared the related TXA_2 analogue (21) from the commercially available

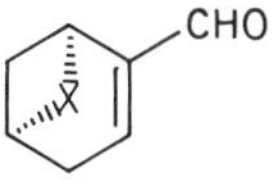

(20) 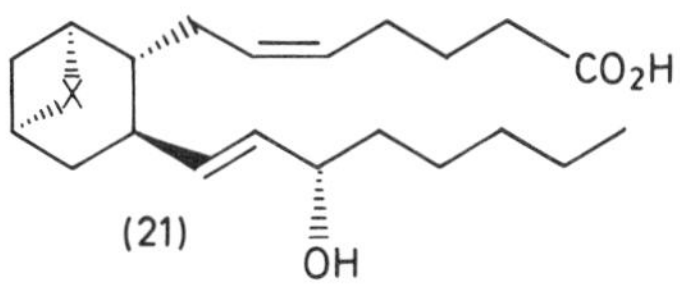 (21)

X = CMe_2

monoterpene (−)-myrtenol (20)[5,6]. Analogue (20) is a TXA_2 antagonist which inhibits vasoconstriction, platelet aggregation and thromboxane synthetase[5].

Several of the TXA_2 analogues that have been prepared seem to possess the hoped-for stability and anti-thrombotic activity. It remains to be seen whether any of these compounds are sufficiently active, specific and non-toxic to be used clinically.

References

1. K.M. MAXEY and G.L. BUNDY, *Tetrahedron Lett.*, 1980, 445.
2. E.J. COREY, J.W. PONDER and P. ULRICH, *Tetrahedron Lett.*, 1980, 137.
3. S. OHUCHIDA, N. HAMANAKA and M. HIYASHI, *Tetrahedron Lett.*, 1979, 3661.
4. K.C. NICOLAOU, R.L. MAGOLDA and D.A. CLAREMON, *J. Am. chem. Soc.*, 1980, **102,** 1404.
5. K.C. NICOLAOU, R.L. MAGOLDA, J.B. SMITH, D. AHARONY, E.F. SMITH and A.M. LEFER, *Proc. natn. Acad. Sci. U.S.A.*, 1979, **76,** 2566.
6. For a different synthesis of 21, *see* M.F. Ansell, M.P.L. Caton, M.N. Palfreyman, K.A.J. Stuttle, *Tetrahedron Lett.*, 1979, 4497.

Index

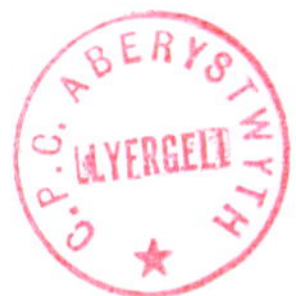